# GLENN LAVERACK

# PUBLIC HEALTH

## POWER, EMPOWERMENT AND PROFESSIONAL PRACTICE

### 3rd edition

First published 2005
Second edition 2009

This edition published 2016 by
PALGRAVE

Palgrave in the UK is an imprint of Macmillan Publishers Limited, registered in England, company number 785998, of 4 Crinan Street, London, N1 9XW.

Palgrave Macmillan in the US is a division of St Martin's Press LLC, 175 Fifth Avenue, New York, NY 10010.

Palgrave is a global imprint of the above companies and is represented throughout the world.

Palgrave® and Macmillan® are registered trademarks in the United States, the United Kingdom, Europe and other countries.

ISBN 978–1–137–54603–6

This book is printed on paper suitable for recycling and made from fully managed and sustained forest sources. Logging, pulping and manufacturing processes are expected to conform to the environmental regulations of the country of origin.

A catalogue record for this book is available from the British Library.

A catalog record for this book is available from the Library of Congress.

Printed in China

# CONTENTS

# LIST OF TABLES, FIGURES AND BOXES

## Tables

## Figures

## Boxes

# ACKNOWLEDGEMENTS

I would like to acknowledge the many people with whom I have had the privilege of working and exchanging ideas during the course of writing the third edition. I would like to thank the publishers for supporting a third edition of the book and to Kristine Crondahl for her comments on Roma migrants.

To Elizabeth, Ben, Holly and Rebecca for their continued love and patience.

# AN OVERVIEW OF THE BOOK

The 3rd edition of the book has four main purposes:

1  to provide the reader with a theoretical understanding of the concepts of power, powerlessness and empowerment in public health programmes in Chapters 1–3
2  to introduce the reader to practical approaches for helping individuals, groups and communities to become empowered in Chapters 4–8
3  to provide the reader with a practical means to measure and visually represent community empowerment in Chapter 9
4  to bring together the main themes of the book and to discuss what the future will have to look like to be more successful in achieving empowerment goals in public health in Chapter 10.

## Chapter 1    Public health practice in context

Chapter 1 provides an introduction to the evolution of empowerment within public health practice, the different roles of the Practitioner and the sometimes problematic relationship that they have with their clients and with other professionals. Chapter 1 introduces the reader to the influence of bureaucratic settings, in which most Practitioners work, and an introduction to how our professional interpretation of public health is a function of our understanding of the concept of health.

## Chapter 2    Power and empowerment

Chapter 2 moves the reader into the territory of how power, powerlessness and empowerment are central to public health practice. The purpose is to allow the reader to better understand complex concepts and the ways in which they interact in practice. Chapter 2 also discusses activism and the relationship that activists have with public health practice.

## Chapter 3    Empowerment and public health programming

Chapter 3 includes a discussion of the tensions that exist in public health programming between 'top-down' and 'bottom-up' approaches and a means to resolve this issue through 'parallel-tracking'. Chapter 3 also discusses the importance of needs assessment and introduces contemporary approaches for the mapping of needs within communities in a programme context.

## Chapter 4   Helping individuals to become empowered

Chapter 4 addresses how Practitioners can better work with individuals to help them to use their sense of autonomy to overcome powerlessness. Chapter 4 also discusses how Practitioners can become more effective communicators, learn to listen, develop a dialogue and help others to reduce harm or to take a moral stance.

## Chapter 5   Patient empowerment

Chapter 5 addresses the contemporary field of patient empowerment, the importance of the professional–patient relationship and the role that advocacy, networks and action groups can play in public health. Chapter 5 also discusses the power of professional language and how this can influence the professional–patient relationship.

## Chapter 6   Helping groups to be more critical

Chapter 6 provides an introduction to working with groups as an important means to help others to become more critically aware of their circumstances. Group work offers the opportunity for people to find a 'voice', to develop their skills and to work with others to achieve their goals. Chapter 6 discusses participatory approaches that can be used to help groups to be more critical, including photo-voice, lay epidemiology, health literacy and strategies for collective decision making.

## Chapter 7   Helping communities to become empowered

Chapter 7 addresses those aspects of empowerment that enhance the ability of communities to better organize and mobilize themselves towards gaining power. Chapter 7 clarifies the concept of 'community' and offers a five-point framework for helping people to become collectively empowered. Chapter 7 also discusses the role of health social movements in public health practice.

## Chapter 8   Helping migrant populations to become empowered

Chapter 8 takes the discussion of helping communities further to examine how Practitioners can work with marginalized and migrant populations with a focus on the needs of Roma. The importance of considering the difference of social and cultural perceptions of power and empowerment and how to resolve conflict in a programme context are also discussed.

## Chapter 9   The measurement and visual representation of community empowerment

Chapter 9 discusses the means of collecting and analysing qualitative information as an important professional competence and for the measurement of community empowerment. The measurement and visual representation of this concept is discussed, with examples of using the domains approach and the spider web configuration in different cultural contexts in public health practice.

## Chapter 10   Public health, power and empowerment

Chapter 10 discusses what the future of public health will have to look like in order to be more successful in achieving empowerment goals. To do this, public health will have to find better ways of engaging with communities to share their priorities and to include them as an asset in the programme, systematically building community capacity, developing more flexible funding mechanisms and being creative to scale-up successful local initiatives.

# 1

# PUBLIC HEALTH PRACTICE IN CONTEXT

## Introduction

Public health practice aims to promote health, prevent disease, treat illnesses, prolong valued life, care for the infirm and provide health care services. Traditionally, such goals have been used to curb the spread of infectious diseases to protect the well-being of the general population (Baggott, 2000). More recently the emphasis has shifted to chronic disease prevention interventions and to changing people's behaviours so that they will adopt a healthier lifestyle. Public health practice also has a broader role – the reduction of social injustice and inequalities in health.

The term 'public health' is used to cover a number of specialist areas, including environmental health, nursing and health promotion. The different interests within public health help to shape what it looks like and the directions it takes as a professional practice. These interests have to compete for limited resources and influence within the framework of national policies. Not surprisingly, public health remains a complex term given the wide range of competing perspectives, priorities and services that it strives to deliver, and power and empowerment are key concepts in a practice that is closely connected to the political context.

In practice, public health still belongs primarily to people employed in the health sector, in the sense that it provides these workers with some conceptual models, professional legitimacy and resources. These people may be titled 'public health promoters' or 'health practitioners', while many more who look to the idea of public health occupy jobs such as nursing and medical practice. In this book, I refer to these people as the 'Practitioner(s)'.

As a profession, public health is largely controlled by government and private sector agencies who employ Practitioners to deliver programmes that are designed to improve or maintain the health of individuals, groups and communities. Professional bodies within public health are expected to display specialization of knowledge, technical competence, responsibility and service delivery. Professionalism is attained through educational qualifications, specialized training, membership in professional associations and the inclusion of professional codes of practice including standards of competence (Turner and Samson, 1995).

## Public health practitioners

Public health practitioners are employed to deliver information, resources and services and are often seen as outside agent by the people who are their clients. Public health always entails some power relationship between different stakeholders, primarily between Practitioners and their clients. I use the term 'clients' to cover the range of people who

1

act as the recipients of the information, resources and services being delivered to promote health, for example, pregnant women, school children, patients or newly arrived migrants. I intentionally use the terms 'Practitioners' and 'clients' in this book to help to demonstrate the unbalanced power relationship that exists in public health practice.

One role of the Practitioner has traditionally been as an enforcer of public health legislation, for example, the Environmental Health Officer or 'Sanitary Policeman'. This role has helped to establish the image of some Practitioners as having power over their clients, through the use of legislation. The role has been supported by much of the work of environmental health departments that are concerned with inspection, licensing, complaint investigations and legal proceedings. An enforcement of the wide range of public health, health protection and food safety legislation by these Practitioners has been seen to be necessary to maintain a healthy and safe environment in different settings. Settings are a place or social context in which people engage in daily activities and in which environmental, organizational and personal factors can interact to affect people's health and well-being. Settings can normally be identified as having physical boundaries, a range of people with defined roles and an organizational structure, and include schools, workplaces, hospitals and prisons (Naidoo and Wills, 2009).

Another role of the Practitioner has been concerned with education, training and specialist services, for example, as that of a nurse providing skills and advice to young mothers at an antenatal group. This role has helped to broaden the image of the Practitioner as a health professional with access to superior technical resources and knowledge.

There is a further role, one that is complementary to the role as an enforcer, educator and technical specialist. It is an important role that has been largely overlooked because many Practitioners do not fully understand how their day-to-day work can help others to empower themselves. One of the main tensions that Practitioners face in an empowering approach to public health practice is whether their clients actually want to be empowered. Public health practice is traditionally professionally led; for example, it is the Practitioner, or the agency that employs them, that selects the clients and the methods to be used in a programme. The initiation of the empowerment process and the enthusiasm for its direction is also often led by the Practitioner. This is contradictory to an empowering approach in which the issue to be addressed and the means of reaching an empowered solution are based on the needs of the client and not the Practitioner. Some clients may not want to be empowered. People, especially if they have lived in powerless circumstances, may feel that they do not have the right or do not possess the motivation to empower themselves. Other individuals and groups such as the mentally ill or people with an addiction may not have the ability to organize and mobilize themselves. What must be remembered is that power cannot be given to people but must be gained by those who want it. The choice to be empowered essentially rests with the individual or group and the role of the Practitioner is to encourage her or his clients to take greater responsibility and control over their lives. For those people who cannot, or who refuse to, take responsibility, public health practice may have to intervene and resort to other means, for example, policy and legislation, to protect the health of the general population from the spread of an infectious disease.

In this book I argue that Practitioners can, and often do, play an important role in facilitating change in their clients, either on a one-to-one basis or through working with groups and communities. Practitioners, who are in a position of relative power, work to help their clients, who are in a relatively powerless position, by providing resources and skills, education and advisory services and by using their professional influence to legitimize the concerns of others. To achieve this, Practitioners may have to work across sectors and with different agencies, both public and private, if they are to develop effective strategies. However, some Practitioners may feel powerlessness in their own work setting, and in Chapter 4 I discuss ways in which Practitioners can overcome powerlessness in a professional context. Practitioners must also be flexible in their approach to working with clients whose abilities have to be developed. The Practitioner may be initially tempted not to involve their clients and may undertake the responsibility of planning and design. This is usually to ensure that programmes are in place in time to meet deadlines. However, participation can be compromised and in the longer term the programme has far less chance of success if the clients are not actively involved.

People can become involved in a more meaningful way in public health programmes by taking part in decision making. The role of the Practitioner shifts to becoming an 'enabler', gaining the trust of and establishing common ground with their clients, which is crucial to the process of empowerment. While Practitioners cannot be expected to have an influence on transforming power relationships across all sectors and at all levels of their everyday work, there are two key areas in which they do have an important role:

1  Practitioners are involved in influencing policies and practices that affect health, from the national to the community level, for example, through their expert power in meetings, technical advisory groups and committees. In order to influence policy and practice, Practitioners need to have a better understanding of the meaning of power and how their relationships with different clients are understood and appropriately acted upon by the profession.

2  In most democratic countries, the process of collective action is used to bring about social and political change through influencing policies. These changes are achieved through the legitimate action of individuals who use their decision making power, for example, to lobby, protest and vote. Practitioners, in their day-to-day work, can help their clients by using their influence to advocate on behalf of others. Participation in groups and organizations is often the first tangible step towards becoming involved in a more collective and organized context, for example, in community-based organizations. This also provides the Practitioner with an opportunity to directly help others to increase their knowledge, skills and competencies more effectively at the collective level.

## The evolution of empowerment in public health practice

Empowerment is defined here as a process by which people are able to gain or seize control over decisions and resources that influence their lives. In the United Kingdom, for example, this concept evolved in public health as an important ideology in the mid-nineteenth century. The political liberalism of the Victorian period led to the creation of many pressure groups, such as the Health of Towns Associations, with a concern for equity and social justice. These pressure groups, with the assistance of key public health reformers such as Edwin Chadwick, were active in mobilizing the middle classes, who in turn had an influence on the press and on the government. This is called the 'sanitation phase' and was a period that through influential reformers and collective action resulted in the government passing key public health legislation such as the 1833 Factories Act and the 1848 Public Health Act (Baggott, 2000). However, these actions were also influenced by the desire of the government to reduce its own responsibilities and to improve the efficiency of the nation's workforce. Public health reform was as much due to the discourse of economic production as it was to the discourse of empowerment and to good governance. During the second phase, occupying the first half of the twentieth century, the growing status of the medical profession added to the political influence of the public health lobby. Consequently, the emphasis was on a public health practice dominated by a bio-medical model and a focus on the absence of disease and illness.

Internationally, it was not until the 1960s and 1970s that empowerment became part of the discourse, stemming from a growing body of 'new knowledge' that sought to challenge conventional thinking. Within public health, the discourse broadened from the bio-medical model to include a behavioural and lifestyle component. The main reasons for this change in thinking were an increase in the role of chronic degenerative diseases, such as heart disease, as the leading causes of morbidity and mortality. These chronic diseases involve the interplay of different determinants over time, such as smoking, lack of exercise and a poor diet, and have become synonymous with an unhealthy lifestyle. At the time public health was closely associated with health education and placed an emphasis on the responsibility of the individual and on a 'victim-blaming' philosophy rather than on collective action and social equity. This made people feel guilty about their poor state of health even though some factors were beyond their control, for example, being made unemployed.

The demands for social justice in the challenge to improve health was increasingly recognized and became the subject of professional discourse, for example, at the 30th World Health Assembly, held in Geneva in May 1977, which set the target of health for all by the year 2000. The following year, an international conference on primary health care in Alma Ata in the former USSR endorsed this target and strongly affirmed the World Health Organization's (WHO) definition of health (World Health Organization, 1986), noting that it was a fundamental human right. The Alma Ata Declaration of 1978 recognized that the gross inequalities in the health status between and within countries were unacceptable and identified primary health care as the key to attaining health for all by the year 2000. The declaration recognized that people must be actively involved in the process of development and went beyond participation to imply that empowerment is a necessary component of primary health care and public health (World Health Organization, 1978).

The Alma Ata Declaration does not use the term 'empowerment' but many of its points imply involvement by individuals and the community. This is in part a reflection of the discourse in the early 1970s when the concept of empowerment had not become fully legitimized. The concept of community participation was viewed as a means to target people as beneficiaries of development by involving them in the process. The discourse argued that participation would allow local knowledge and needs to be incorporated into a programme and would give people more control in decision making. In practice, this depends on the power relationship between Practitioners and their clients. Practitioners can use their power, for example, to take a paternalistic stance and to coerce others into the programme rather than to encourage them to actively participate.

Since the early 1980s there has been a shift within public health towards greater participation embodied in the socio-environmental approach, which was guided by key strategic documents such as the Ottawa Charter for Health Promotion (World

Health Organization, 1986). Another key factor was an increased awareness of growing inequalities in health status between different social groups and the narrowness of the focus on individual behaviour that ignored the psychosocial and physical environments, community and culture. It was recognized that the individualistic nature of public health campaigns did not recognize the social and environmental contexts in which personal behaviours are embedded. At the same time, many pressure groups and health social movements challenged the notion of the medical and behavioural approaches to health and raised concerns for social justice and environmental sustainability.

## Power and public health practice

Public health practice is largely carried out through bureaucratic settings. The bureaucratic setting consists of a number of distinctive positions of power with specialist duties that are usually formally defined. The officials who hold these positions of power are recruited according to specific rules and their employment is usually based on a system of salaries. Power is hierarchically top-down and the official is expected to act in accordance with, and without challenging, the instructions descending from their superiors (Turner and Samson, 1995). Examples of highly bureaucratic and hierarchical public health organizations include government departments and hospitals. Positioning oneself within the hierarchy of a bureaucratic setting provides professional legitimacy, expert power and status. This is achieved not necessarily because that person has particular expertise but because the institutionalization of the position creates the idea that she or he is an expert.

### Using professional power in public health

If it is true that public health is a bureaucratic activity, carried out by or within governmental organizations or government-funded agencies, it is also true that many of these organizations remain chained to traditional ways of thinking and acting, ways which can inhibit the effective inclusion of empowering approaches. Studies of both governmental and non-governmental agencies have found that the concepts of empowerment used in policy and practice are often quite different. Despite the intent to empower communities, the agencies and their staff tended to retain control over programming rather than relinquishing power to others. The agencies operated within a contradiction between discourse and practice: many Practitioners continued to exert power over the community through top-down programming while at the same time using an emancipatory discourse (Laverack, 1999). To build a more empowering practice, public health must redress the constraints placed on the profession by its bureaucratic nature and by others who do not share an ideology of empowerment. Before Practitioners can empower others they must first be themselves empowered and understand the sources of their own power. Within a bureaucratic setting, for example, a hospital, a community of both patients and staff, both must be empowered and this includes feeling valued and having the resources, skills and knowledge to empower others (Kendall, 1998).

But governments and the bureaucracies that they create, at least in democratic countries, are not monolithic entities. Not only are there often contradictions between the policies and actions of different government agencies but different Practitioners with differing ideas often exist and work together. Practitioners working in large bureaucratic settings can find their professional autonomy being undermined by the hierarchical structure of rules and lines of control. Professional groups can also become fragmented into sub-groups or else their power base is encroached upon by para-professional groups. These circumstances actually present opportunities for an empowering practice to develop within even the largest, most rigid bureaucracies. To take advantage of these opportunities public health agencies must understand how to address imbalances in the power relationships in their structures at all levels, from the top tiers of policy and planning to the Practitioners working at the interface with the community. It is precisely this type of fundamental issue that must be addressed if Practitioners are to engage in an empowering approach in their daily work.

In a professional context the key question is: Do Practitioners really want to help to empower people or simply to change their behaviour? The latter has traditionally been the most popular choice and the difference between an empowering approach and a coercive approach has been in the method used. If the method is directive, top-down and controlled by an outside agent, it is less likely to be empowering. If it facilitates a process of needs identification and actions based on the concerns of the individual or community, using strategies to build capacity, it will have a much better chance of being empowering. Practitioners must make the decision to empower themselves, to gain the necessary skills and knowledge, if they are really committed to an approach that will empower others. Empowerment approaches are also dependent on funding and on there being a political will to implement them. This may be problematic when the goal of the people who are involved in community empowerment is to bring about a change in the political order and to challenge the very status of the agencies that support their continuation. This is a power relationship that must be equalized and which is a central theme of this book.

## Public health practice and the interpretation of health

The multiplicity of meanings assigned to public health is also a function of the multiplicity of meanings assigned to our understandings of health. In practice, it can be useful to consider the distinction between official understandings, those used by public health professionals, and lay understandings, the perceptions held by those who are usually the recipients of health interventions, the public. Official definitions of health can differ significantly from lay definitions but both are ideal types and in practice coexist and inform one another.

Practitioners have largely used official interpretations because these are easier to define and measure, rather than lay interpretations of health, which are subjective, being based on the experiences of the individual. In particular, the bio-medical interpretation of health has established itself as the most dominant official interpretation. It is the medical profession which has been the champion of this model of health, based on the absence of disease and illness, and upon which other health professions have modelled themselves, including the field of public health.

The bio-medical model evolved as a result of scientific discoveries and technological advances in the eighteenth and nineteenth centuries, which led to a greater understanding of the structure and functioning of the human body. As knowledge and understanding increased, health took on an increasingly mechanistic meaning. The body was viewed as a machine that needed to be fixed. A professional split between the body and mind developed; the body and its physical illness was the responsibility of physicians while psychologists and psychiatrists looked after the psyche and its illnesses. However, the focus remained on the external causes of ill health and was reinforced by the constant threat of disease and death from epidemics such as polio and scarlet fever (Laverack, 2009).

The official interpretations of health can be divided into two main types: those which define health negatively and those which adopt a more positive stance. There are two main ways of viewing health negatively. The first equates with the absence of disease or bodily abnormality, the second with the absence of illness or the feelings of anxiety, pain or distress that may or may not accompany the disease. Some people may be diseased without knowing it and are unaware of their condition until they start to suffer pain and discomfort, when the person is said to be ill. Negative definitions of health emphasize the absence of disease or illness and are the basis for the medical model. A number of problems have been raised concerning the negative definition of health. In particular, the notion of pathology implies that certain universal norms exist against which an individual can be assessed when making a judgement as to whether or not they are healthy. This assumes that such standards actually exist in human anatomy and physiology.

## The World Health Organization's definition of health

The first modern positive definition of health came in 1948 when the World Health Organization (WHO) stated that health was 'a state of complete physical, social and mental well-being, and not merely the absence of disease or infirmity' (Jackson et al., 1989). Physical well-being is concerned with concepts such as the proper functioning of the body, biological normality, physical fitness and capacity to perform tasks. Social well-being includes interpersonal relationships as well as wider social issues such as marital satisfaction, employability and social inclusion. The role of relations, the family and status at work are important to a person's social well-being. Mental well-being involves concepts such as self-efficacy, subjective well-being and social inclusion, and is the ability of people to adapt to their environment and the society in which they function.

The WHO definition has become one of the most influential and commonly used in public health and for that reason its origins, which are set in the context of empowerment, are worth exploring, and are explained in Box 1.1. The WHO definition of health, as an ideal state of physical, social and mental well-being, has been criticized for not taking other dimensions of health into account, namely the emotional and spiritual aspects of health (Ewles and Simnett, 2003). The definition has also been criticized for viewing health as a state or product rather than as a dynamic relationship, a capacity, a potential or a process and for not clarifying how to define or measure its components.

## Box 1.1 The origins of the WHO definition of health

The WHO definition was written soon after the Second World War by an official who had spent his time working in the Resistance. He had come to this definition from his experience and explained that he had never felt healthier than during that terrible period: for he daily worked for goals about which he cared passionately, he was certain that should he be killed in his dangerous work, his family would be cared for by the network of Resistance workers. It was under these circumstances that he felt most

*(Continued)*

healthy, most alive. The definition of health was developed by a person who was passionately involved with others to change social and political structures. In other words, they were involved in taking control over those things which affect their lives and by doing so empowered themselves and improved their own health and well-being as well as that of others with whom they associated (Jackson et al., 1989).

## The subjective view of health

The way in which people interpret the meaning of their own health is a personal and sometimes unique experience. Health is a subjective concept and its interpretation is relative to the environment and culture in which people are situated, and therefore health can mean different things to different people. Many people define health in functional terms, for example, by their ability to carry out certain roles and responsibilities rather than the absence of disease. People may be willing to bear the discomfort and pain of an illness because it does not outweigh the inconvenience, loss of control or financial cost of having the condition treated (Laverack, 2009). This subjective view of health raises the issue of radical relativism, which maintains that the only true reality is the unique experience of the individual. While it is important to understand individual feelings and experiences about health, there may be others that are common to particular groups. Inter-subjectivity is a concept used to overcome the limitations of radical relativism. It claims that any given person's understanding of the world is unique but because it is constructed from a field of more or less common social meanings and experiences, communication between people is possible. In other words, the meanings we create of our own experiences of health overlap sufficiently to allow us to communicate and share these experiences with others. However, this may not necessarily lead to a positive health outcome; for example, the biological and behavioural traits associated with obesity appear to be spread through social ties. People who experience the weight gain of others in their social ties may then more readily accept weight gain in themselves because people's perceptions of their own risk of illness depends on the people around them (Christakis and Fowler, 2007).

Self-esteem is also a social phenomenon and a person's self-regard and sense of coherence is not grounded in 'the self', but in relation to friends, family, colleagues, communities and in the settings in which they live and work. Social support is therefore generally accepted as having a beneficial effect on health, both at an individual and at a collective level; for example, by sharing problems people are better able to cope with stressful events. Social support is connected to other similar overlapping concepts such as social capital, social inclusiveness, social exclusiveness and salutogenesis (see Chapter 5). These concepts fundamentally address a sense of connection to a 'community' and the involvement and trust between its members manifested through customs, rituals and traditional groupings.

Some commentators have concluded that it is futile to try to define health because it is too subjective and complex and it is better framed within the context of the services offered and that society can afford (Jadad and O'Grady, 2008). In practice, public health programming is increasingly concerned with accountability to funders, effectiveness and value for money. Budgetary constraints, competition for funding and priorities for health have also had a strong influence on the way in which health has been interpreted. Public health has, for the time being, decided to take the pragmatic view that whatever interpretation of health is used it must be measurable and accountable; otherwise programmes will be in jeopardy of being unable to justify their economic and quantifiable effectiveness. Health is considered to be a means to an end that can be expressed in functional terms as a resource which permits people to lead an individually, socially and economically productive life. This being the case, the measurement of health has focused on a bio-medical approach that is concerned with demonstrating a relationship between a health status measure and a health-related behaviour such as smoking and lung cancer. The boundaries for practice and discourse have consequently been defined by the interpretations of illness and disease rather than by the way in which most people generally view or feel that they need to maintain their own health.

Next, Chapter 2 moves the reader into the territory of how power, powerlessness and empowerment are central to public health practice. The purpose is to make these complex concepts, and the way in which they interact, more understandable in a practical sense.

# 2

# POWER AND EMPOWERMENT

Power and empowerment are central to public health, and yet many Practitioners still do not fully understand how these concepts can be applied as part of their everyday work. This can lead to a contradiction between the professional discourse and practice: many Practitioners continue to exert control over their clients through 'top-down' programmes, while at the same time using an emancipatory ideology and language. Plainly put, many Practitioners do not have a clear understanding of how their work can help to empower individuals, groups and communities. However, to blame the Practitioner would be to underestimate the important role that they have in empowering their clients. For public health to use an empowering approach, Practitioners must understand how power is an integral part of their working relationship and how this can transform what they do to help others gain more control over their lives and health.

## What is power?

The most common interpretation of power is in the form of hard power, in which one person has control over others. It is the capacity of some to produce intended and foreseen effects on others (Wrong, 1988, p. 2). Power can also be a social phenomenon: one that can be vested in groups and communities that are better able to identify and control the basis of their power. In contrast to hard power, soft power is the ability to obtain what one wants through indirect and long-term actions, such as co-option and attraction. The difference is therefore that hard power achieves compliance through direct and coercive methods and by compelling others to do what you want them to do, whether they want to do it or not. The purpose of soft power is to persuade others to voluntarily do what you want them to do but to avoid conflict. The primary currencies of soft power are values, culture, policies and institutions, agenda control and the extent to which these are able to attract or repel others. The phrase 'you are either with us or against us' is an exercise in soft power, since no explicit threat is included, although there is an implied threat that direct economic or military sanctions would likely follow. The success of soft power can depend on one person's reputation as well as on the flow of information. The media is regularly identified as a source of soft power, as is the spread of a national language, or a particular set of normative values (Gallarotti, 2011). An example of soft power is moral suasion (see Chapter 4): the use of moral principles to influence individuals and groups to change their practices, beliefs and actions (Berridge, 2007). Because soft power has appeared as an alternative to hard power, it is often embraced by ethically minded scholars and policy makers, but it has also been criticized as being ineffective and too difficult to distinguish from the effects of other factors.

To exercise choice is the simplest form of power. This may involve the trivial health choices of everyday life, such as which brand of toothpaste to buy, or the more critical choices, such as whether or not to stop smoking. Practitioners should recognize that the rhetoric of choice can become an excuse for health professionals to avoid difficult issues and to transfer blame. The trivial choices should not cloud the more critical issues where the powerless have no choice, for example, promoting an active lifestyle when poor people cannot afford to do more exercise or do not have the time or a supportive environment in which to do so. Box 2.1 provides an example of how Asian women got involved in choices about improving their lifestyle and levels of physical activity in Liverpool in the UK.

## Box 2.1 The Asian women's swimming project

The Asian Health Forum in Liverpool, England, identified a large number of cases of depression and social exclusion in the area through discussions among Asian women. The women suggested more opportunities to do exercise and to meet other women, and a health worker was asked by them to approach a local leisure centre about the possibility of arranging swimming lessons solely for these women. This would ensure privacy, for example, windows would be blacked out and the lessons would be run only by other women. The agreement between the Asian women and the leisure centre allowed them to organize weekly lessons and to secure funding for a female instructor. The swimming lessons were popular and timings had to be reorganized to avoid conflict with other pool activities and to accommodate the participation of the young children of the women. The lessons continued throughout the summer with about 20 women attending per session, and slowly the interest of the women moved to other sports activities (Jones and Sidell, 1997, p. 41). This model for promoting physical activity and increasing the choices available to Asian women has been successfully replicated elsewhere.

To the extent that our personal choices constrain those of others, power can become an exercise of control. People with the ability to control decisions at the political and economic level can condition and constrain the ability of people to exercise choice at the individual and group level. People may have control over others but at the same time can be constrained and influenced by those who have power over them.

# Three variations of power

To better understand how power can be exercised in both the sharing of control with others and the use of control to exert influence over others, it is helpful for Practitioners to consider three different variations: 'power-from-within'; 'power-over'; and 'power-with'.

# Power-from-within

Power-from-within can be described as a personal power or some inner sense of strength, self-discipline or self-esteem. Power-from-within is also known as individual, personal or psychological empowerment: the means of gaining (a sense of) control over one's life (Rissel, 1994) with the goal of increasing feelings of value and a greater sense of control. Thomas Wartenberg, a writer on the different forms of power, argues that even in the most male-dominated, controlling society women have power: their power-from-within. Likewise, Western feminist theory claims that although women are not socially dominant, they do have special skills and inner strengths that have enabled them to act in invaluable ways. Once one has accepted this, Wartenberg's (1990, p. 188) argument that 'women both have and lack power in a male dominated society' can be seen to contain an important insight into power-from-within. Individuals can become more powerful from within and do not necessarily have to accumulate money, status or authority. However, the individualization of this concept can lead to public health approaches that aim to increase the notion of 'self', for example, in assertiveness classes, ignoring how another form of power, power-over, can constrain experiences of control in people's everyday lives (Laverack, 2004).

## Power-over

Power-over describes social relationships in which one party is made to do what another party wishes them to do despite their resistance, and even if it may not be in their best interests. Starhawk (1990, p. 9) describes power-over in its rawest form as 'the power of the prison guard, of the gun, power that is ultimately backed by force'. However, the exercise of power-over does not always have to be negative; for example, legislation to control the spread of diseases through quarantine or to impose fines for unhygienic behaviour, such as for food handlers not washing their hands, are considered as healthy power-over. Power-over can take different forms depending on how it is used to exert control or to affect the actions of others, for example, dominance, or the direct power to control people's choices, usually by force or its threat. The resources that Practitioners may bring to bear on their clients have been identified as six bases of power-over: coercion; reward; legitimacy; expertise; reference and information. To put the six bases of power-over into a public health context, I use the example of a breast feeding intervention:

1  In **coercive power**, the Practitioner may bring about negative consequences or punishment for the mother if she does not comply; for example, using disapproving language towards her for not breast feeding her child.
2  In **reward power**, the Practitioner may bring about positive consequences for the mother upon compliance; for example, by praising her for breast feeding and keeping her child clean.
3  **Legitimate power** stems from the mother accepting a social role relationship with the Practitioner, a structural relationship which grants him/her the right to prescribe behaviour for the mother, while the mother accepts an obligation to comply with the requests of the Practitioner. The mother accepts the legitimate professional position of a nurse and listens to and then carries out his/her advice on breast feeding.
4  **Expert power** stems from the mother attributing superior knowledge and ability to the Practitioner; for example, the phrase 'Doctor knows best' illustrates the expert power relationship between the patient and doctor.
5  **Referent power** stems from an identification of the mother with the Practitioner: a feeling of communality, similarity and mutual interest. The mother then gets some satisfaction from believing and complying in a manner consistent with the beliefs,

attitudes and behaviours of the Practitioner. This may be based on the gender, social class, ethnicity or empathy shown by a nurse Practitioner towards the breast feeding mother.

6 **Informational power** is based on the explicit information communicated to the mother from the Practitioner, a persuasive communication that will convince the mother that the recommended behaviour is indeed in the mother's best interests; for example, advice on child spacing, including breast feeding. Informational power is commonly used in health education; however, it is important to note that the phrase 'Knowledge is power' can be misleading and is not necessarily correct. New knowledge without the means to carry out the prescribed actions can simply lead to people having a greater sense of powerlessness. For example, informing the breast feeding mother to eat healthy foods for the benefit of herself and her child when she cannot afford to buy these products can lead to her having a greater sense of a lack of control in her life (Raven and Litman-Adizes, 1986).

## Hegemonic power

Hegemony is the ability of a dominant group to control the actions and behaviours of others by intense persuasion and exploitation and to control people's choices through economic relations, in which those who control capital also have control over those who do not (Wrong, 1988). Hegemonic power is that form of power-over that is internalized and structured into our everyday lives and taken for granted. To Michel Foucault, a prominent theorist and commentator on power, the only form of resistance to hegemonic power is a concealment of one's life from those in authority and the judgements that it can create (Foucault, 1979). A practical example of this is a single parent mother living in government-funded housing hiding her sick child from a health visitor or lowering the toilet seat to avoid suspicion that she is cohabitating with a man. Persons living in conditions of hegemonic power-over, of oppression and exploitation, internalize these conditions as being their personal responsibility. This internalization increases their own self-blame and decreases their self-esteem. One of the subtle, but common, ways in which Practitioners participate in hegemonic power is when they continually impose their expert ideas of what are important health problems without actually listening to what their clients think are important for their health.

The rise of the medical profession has been successful in maintaining its position of dominance within a bureaucratic hierarchy by controlling access to health care delivery. This has been termed the 'hegemony of the medical profession'. The medical profession has formed itself as a powerful professional pressure group and although not a complete monopoly, because of the growth of other health professions, has been granted considerable control to maintain self-regulation and clinical autonomy in its work. This dominance, for example, has been blamed for the historical subordination of the nursing profession and has been seen as a key challenge to nurse empowerment (Kendall, 1998). Much of the power held by the medical profession is supported by the public, who expect confidentiality in the special relationship that they hold with their doctor. The medical profession is also dependent on alliances with other health professionals, the government, the private sector, science and activists. It has been careful to create an alignment between both professional and public interests, for example, in regard to the under-resourcing of the UK National Health Service, long waiting times for treatment and the unacceptable demands placed on hospital staff. This professional dominance has also been paralleled with an increase in the legitimacy of medical knowledge, urbanization, the expansion of health insurance and the growth of bureaucratic settings, such as hospitals as centres for 'professional excellence' (Turner and Samson, 1995). Despite the dominance of the medical profession, there have been challenges to its expert wisdom from, for example, the health social movements (see Chapter 7) and through lay epidemiology (Chapter 6).

## Power-with

Power-with describes a different set of social relationships in which power-over is deliberately used to increase other people's power, rather than to dominate or exploit them. Power-over transforms to power-with only when it has effectively reached its end: when the submissive person in the relationship has accrued enough power-from-within to exercise his or her own choices. The person with the power-over chooses not to dominate but to begin a discussion that will increase the other's level of control. The Practitioner offers advice to their clients in the identification and resolution of problems to help develop their power-from-within. The transformative use of power-over also demands a great deal of self-vigilance by all persons in the relationship, but in particular by the initially more dominant person: the Practitioner. If not, the relationship can remain as power-over; for example, using the different instruments of social power discussed above: referent power or mentoring that does not try to come to completion can become charismatic authority or 'guruization'; and legitimate or expert power that does not acknowledge that others in the relationship may have their own expertise can lead to a patronizing inducement of dependency.

## Powerlessness

Powerlessness, or the absence of power, whether imagined or real, is an individual concept with the expectancy that the behaviour of a person cannot determine the outcomes they seek. It combines an attitude of self-blame, a sense of generalized distrust, a feeling of alienation from resources for social influence, an experience of disenfranchisement and economic vulnerability and a sense of hopelessness in gaining social and political influence (Kieffer, 1984). The process by which people may perceive themselves as being powerless is described in Box 2.2.

---

**Box 2.2 Experiencing powerlessness**

The process by which people may perceive themselves as being powerless can begin when individuals and groups living in risk conditions, or who experience inequalities in health (poor housing, unemployment, insanitary conditions), feel distress with the unfairness of their situation (their low status on some hierarchy of power or authority, indicated in part by wealth). These people then internalize this feeling of unfairness as aspects of their own 'badness' or 'failure'. This internalization adds to their distress, if

*(Continued)*

not also to their loss of meaning and purpose, with measurable effects on their bodies such as hypertension (Labonté, 1998). The powerless often experience little leverage on the events and conditions that impinge on their existence, either directly or through access to resources, information and facilities. This situation is made worse when the dominant social discourse on success is competitiveness, individualism and meritocracy, where people are presumed to succeed or fail purely on the basis of their own initiative or ability (Lerner, 1986). This internalization of 'badness' leads to what is described as learned helplessness (Seligman, 1975).

Michael Lerner (1986), a political scientist and psychotherapist, argues that persons living in high-risk conditions, for example, in slum housing, can experience what he named as 'surplus powerlessness'. This is a surplus created by, but distinct from, external or objective conditions of powerlessness. In surplus powerlessness, individuals internalize their objective or external powerlessness and create a potent psychological barrier to empowering action. They do not even engage in activities that meet their real needs. They begin to accept aspects of their world that are self-destructive to their own health and well-being, thinking that these are unalterable features of what they take to be a reality.

Power and powerlessness are relative concepts, as one can have authority or social status by virtue of others not having it. Someone may have authority or status in one situation, relative to others, but not in another situation. Practitioners therefore need to look for, and work from, areas in people's lives in which they are relatively powerful.

## Zero-sum and non-zero-sum

Zero-sum power exists when one can only possess x amount of power to the extent that someone else has the absence of an equivalent amount. It is therefore a 'win/lose' situation. My power-over you plus your absence of that power, equals zero (thus the term, 'zero-sum'). I win and you lose. For you to gain power you must seize it from me. If you can, you win and I lose. Power is used as leverage to raise the position of one person or group, while simultaneously lowering it for another person or group. However, at any one time there will be only so much leverage (wealth, control, resources) possessed within a society. This distribution and the decision making authority that goes with it is zero-sum. At the same time, there are dominant forms of status or privilege, such as class, gender, education and ethnic background, which tend to structure relations in most social situations. Practitioners, in the course of their work, may find it unavoidable to help some people but not others. Public health policy can sometimes place a requirement on Practitioners to work with specific groups, such as the poor, the homeless or the 'unhealthy'. It is based on the interpretation of power as being resource-dependent and reliant on some type of material product. It essentially ignores that power can also be a result of social relations, including the relationship one has with oneself (power-from-within).

There is therefore another important concept of power, one that is regarded not as fixed and finite, but as infinite and expanding. This is the non-zero-sum form of power that is 'win/win', since it is based on the idea that if any one person or group gains, everyone else also gains. Trust, caring and other aspects of our social relationships with one another are examples of non-zero-sum power. To be more empowering in their work, Practitioners should gravitate towards the non-zero-sum formulation. Power is no longer seen as a finite commodity, such as wealth, or as the comparative status and authority that this might confer. Rather, non-zero-sum power takes the form of relationships based on respect, generosity, service to others, a free flow of information and commitment to the ethics of caring and justice. The role of the Practitioner in this construction of power is to use these attributes to engender them in others and to transfer power in part by providing better access to information and resources (Laverack, 2004).

In practice, public health simultaneously involves the zero-sum and non-zero-sum forms of power. Power cannot be given, but communities can be enabled by Practitioners to gain power from others. Practitioners must first identify their own power bases, and then through the professional–client relationship share this power base to enable others to gain control over the influences on their lives and health. For example, the education level and professional training, higher income, expert status and social class, influence over decision makers, familiarity with systems of bureaucracy and control over budget allocations are all forms of Practitioner power bases. Practitioners generally do have more power or a stronger power base than their clients and must understand how to use this to help others to gain power.

## Empowerment: the means to attaining power

Empowerment is the means to attaining power. In the broadest sense it is 'the process by which disadvantaged people work together to increase control over events that determine their lives' (Werner, 1988, p. 1). Most definitions give the term a similarly positive value and embody the notion that empowerment must come from within an individual, group or community. The essence of empowerment is that it cannot be given and must be gained by those who seek it. Those who have power or have access to it, such as Practitioners, and those who want it, such as their clients, must work together to create the conditions necessary to make empowerment in public health possible. In professional practice, this is a mutual role played out by the Practitioner, who can facilitate change, and the clients, who identify and execute the change. However, as discussed above, one must be able to identify one's own power base in order to share it with others. The inability of some Practitioners to identify and use their power base may account for the act of helping others to gain power being neglected in favour of the act of attempting to help others simply through the delivery of information, resources or services.

The concept of empowerment is usually portrayed as existing at one or more levels, namely, individual, family, organizational and community. Christopher Rissel (1994, p. 41) includes a heightened or increased level of psychological (individual) empowerment as a part of community empowerment. He argues that community empowerment includes 'a political action component in which members have actively participated, and the achievement of some redistribution of resources or decision making favourable to the community or group in question'. Barbara Israel and her colleagues (1994) similarly identify psychological and political action as two levels of community empowerment, but include a third, and intermediary, level between them: that of organizational empowerment. An empowered organization is one that is democratically managed; its members share information and control over decisions and are involved in the design, implementation and control of efforts towards goals defined by group consensus. Haynes and Singh (1993) provide a model for 'family empowerment' as a social unit within communities which are able to organize themselves to gain power. This is a common theme in non-westernized societies, where importance is placed on the well-being of social units, such as the family, rather than on the individual. Conversely, public health programmes are very often targeted at the individual; for example, to change behaviour or to increase knowledge. The danger is that this approach can be inappropriately superimposed onto other socio-cultural contexts that focus on the family or community unit rather than on the individual. The family is the core unit of society in these cultural contexts and the purpose of empowerment is to give families, groups and communities more control at the appropriate level so that they can address their own needs.

Community empowerment is an interaction between individual, family and organizational forms of empowerment. It occurs at both an individual and a collective level and is a dynamic process involving continual shifts in power between different individuals and groups in society. Community empowerment is also an outcome, and in this form it can be measured as a redistribution of resources, a decrease in powerlessness or success in achieving greater control (Rappaport, 1985). However, empowerment is most consistently viewed as a process that progresses along a continuum in which people become increasingly better organized towards social and political action and can be measured as a set of organizational factors or domains.

Per-Anders Tengland (2007) concludes from a conceptual analysis of collective empowerment that as an outcome or as a process, it has applicability for creating opportunity to improve health. He believes that the logic for using an empowering approach in public health is justified, because it is based on well-founded theory that has empirical support, and because it is ethically or morally sound to do so. He also recognizes that many Practitioners do not have the knowledge and skills that are required to undertake an empowering approach and raises the issue of adequate training. Practitioners often work with clients from different cultural backgrounds and they need to have a shared understanding of empowerment if they are to use this approach in their everyday work. Training would therefore have to include a better understanding of ourselves as Practitioners, our beliefs and values and to put this into a framework of other social and cultural perceptions of power and empowerment.

## Activism

Activism is action on behalf of a cause: action that goes beyond what is considered to be routine in society (Martin, 2007). What constitutes activism depends on what is conventional in society, as any action is relative to others. In practice, activist organizations employ a combination of both conventional and unconventional strategies to achieve their goals (Laverack, 2013). Activism has an explicit purpose to help to empower others and this is embodied in actions that are typically energetic, passionate, innovative and committed. Activism has played a major role in protecting workers from exploitation, protecting the environment, promoting equality for women and opposing racism. Activism is a dynamic process because organizations can choose to use a variety of tactics, culturally informed and to some extent shaped by local laws, political opportunity, culture and technology. However, activism is not always used positively, as the actions of some minority groups can oppose human rights and the beliefs of the majority.

The types of actions that activist organizations engage in can be broadly sub-divided into two categories: indirect and direct.

1   Indirect actions are non-violent and often require a minimum of effort, including voting, signing a petition, taking part in a 'virtual (online) sit-in' and sending an email to protest your cause.
2   Direct actions can range from peaceful protests to inflicting intentional physical damage on persons and property. The focus is on short-term action, with the primary, and often only, goal being to have an immediate effect. Direct action can be used in a symbolic way to send a message to the general public, and/or to the owners, shareholders and employees of a specific company, and/or to policy makers, about specific grievances.

Direct actions can be further sub-divided into non-violent and violent actions.

2.1   Non-violent actions include protests, picketing, vigils, marches, publicity campaigns and taking legal action. Consumer boycotts are an example of non-violent actions focused on the long-term change of buying habits and the reform of consumer markets. Consumer boycotting was an early tactic of activists to try to punish corporations, but by the 1990s the trend was more towards developing standards and accrediting retail products that would be rewarded by consumers. Concerns were raised that boycotting products may force the people involved in the labour of manufacture to turn to more dangerous sources of income (UNICEF, 2001).
2.2   Violent actions include physical tactics against people or property, placing oneself in a position of manufactured vulnerability to prevent action, such as standing in front of a bulldozer or taking part in an act of civil disobedience.

Health activism involves a challenge to the existing order whenever it is perceived to influence people's health negatively or has led to an injustice or an inequity. The tactics of health activism have continued to evolve along with new developments in technology. Cell phone messaging, for example, is extensively used to communicate and to organize protests. Health activism also continues to raise new issues including sexual harassment, bullying and domestic violence by campaigning about them and by developing techniques to address the inequities that these issues create (Plows, 2007).

Next, Chapter 3 discusses the tensions that exist in public health programming between 'top-down' and 'bottom-up' approaches and offers a way forward to resolve this issue through 'parallel-tracking'. Chapter 3 also discusses the importance of needs assessment and introduces contemporary approaches for the mapping of needs within communities in a public health programme context.

# 3

# EMPOWERMENT AND PUBLIC HEALTH PROGRAMMING

## Introduction

In practice, public health is most commonly implemented as activities set within the context of an intervention, a project or a programme. In this book, I have used the term 'programme' to cover all of these situations. The programme cycle is conventionally managed and monitored by Practitioners and includes a period of identification, design, appraisal, approval, implementation, management and evaluation. The considerations for the programme are documented as an agreement between the different stakeholders, such as a Memorandum of Understanding, or as a technical framework. The purpose is to outline the aims, objectives, inputs, outputs, impact and other details of the programme.

The way in which public health programmes address and define particular needs is one of the most important issues. This can take two main forms: 'top-down' and 'bottom-up'. 'Top-down' describes programmes in which needs assessment comes from the top structures in the system down to the community, defined by the outside agent. 'Bottom-up' is the reverse, in which the community identifies its own needs and communicates these to the top structures. Top-down programming is a manifestation of power-over, in which the Practitioner exercises control of financial and other material resources over the programme. It is a form of dominance in which control is exerted through the design, implementation and evaluation of the programme. I intentionally use the terms top-down and bottom-up in this book because they help to illustrate the power relationship that commonly exists in public health programming: The Practitioner uses their power-over to push down a predefined agenda onto the community with the assumption that this will give them more control. Top-down and bottom-up approaches are ideal types of best practice and demonstrate important differences in relation to programme design, and in Table 3.1 I show the main differences between these two styles in public health.

Public health programmes are typically centred on improving health or preventing disease. This can become problematic when it creates a 'bottom-up versus top-down tension', as communities struggle to get their needs addressed or heard within the programme design. However, at the early stages of the programme cycle, the design stage, there are a number of important considerations such as the time frame, language and terminology and needs assessment that can help to promote greater community involvement.

Too short a time frame, for example, runs the real risk of initiating community-level changes, only to end before such changes have reached a degree of sustainability within the community. The programme should therefore start with realistic community achievable goals that can produce visible successes and in the short term. This is to sustain the interest of the community and to promote the progression onto other initiatives. It is at the design stage that the power relationship is established between the Practitioner and the other stakeholders of the programme, in particular, the intended beneficiaries. During

Table 3.1   The different characteristics of top-down and bottom-up approaches

| Characteristic | Top-down approaches | Bottom-up approaches |
|---|---|---|
| Role of agents | Outside agents define the issue, develop strategies to resolve the issue, involve the community to assist with solving the issue. | Outside agents act to support the community in the identification of issues which are important and relevant to their lives and enable them to develop strategies to resolve these issues. |
| Design | Defined short- to medium-term time frame, budget, stakeholder analysis. | Long term without defined programme time frame. |
| Objectives | Objectives are determined by outside agent and are usually concerned with changing specific behaviours to reduce disease and improve health. | Community identifies objectives which are negotiated with outside agent. These may be concerned with disease and behaviours, but also with community empowerment outcomes and political and social changes. |
| Implementation | Control over decisions essentially rests with outside agent. | Control over decisions is constantly being negotiated. |
| Terminology | Also known as community-based and social planning programmes. | Also known as community empowerment, community development and community capacity-building programmes. |
| Evaluation | Evaluation concerned with targets and outcomes often determined by the outside agents. | Evaluation concerned with process and outcomes and inclusion of the participants. |

Laverack and Labonté (2000, p. 256).

the design phase, Practitioners must be prepared to listen to what people want; they may not necessarily like what they hear, but they must be committed to moving forward by building upon what needs are expressed.

It is important that a programme uses a language and terminology that is understood by all stakeholders. Lay interpretations, for example, of power and empowerment, can be used alongside more technical language so that everyone has a mutual understanding of the programme purpose. Box 3.1 provides an example of the procedure used to develop a working definition of empowerment in a programme in a Fijian context through simple qualitative techniques.

## Box 3.1 Developing a working definition for empowerment

One programme in Fiji used simple qualitative techniques to quickly identify the key local terms for power and empowerment. Unstructured interviews were first used with programme participants to identify the headings for power-over, or lewa, power-from-within and power-with, or kaukauwa. Then through semi-structured interviews the term 'lewa' was further identified to refer to 'chiefly lewa', the control of the village chief and the power-over bestowed at work or in the home. The term kaukauwa is the

(Continued)

closest concept in a Fijian context to empowerment. It refers to community strength and unity, which can be developed and assisted by its members and can be used to describe the right a person has to do something. Chiefly lewa is a state, a status that is bestowed by birthright or by others in an accepted way and is interdependent on the strength or kaukauwa of the community. It is in the interests of the person with the chiefly lewa and the community to maintain and increase the kaukauwa. The relationship is reciprocal and, in this way, the lewa and kaukauwa play an important role in the unity and strength of the community. The kaukauwa may be a mechanism by which the community manage the authority delegated to them by the person with the lewa. It may also be a mechanism used when the community decides to resist and challenge this authority. Although the two terms provide a common understanding, this can depend on how they are used in a programme; for example, the term kaukauwa in the form 'veivakakaukauwataki' suggests action and a process rather than just a concept and would be a more useful term (Laverack, 1998).

## Needs assessment

Needs assessment is used to identify those needs that are reported by an individual, group or community and the resources and outcomes that are required to resolve them (Gilmore, 2011). A needs assessment is a logical starting point of any public health programme because it can include all partners in its design and can build long-term working relationships. Community asset mapping, for example, is an inventory of the strengths of the people, the social interconnections and networks and how these can be accessed. This is important because the opportunities for public health programmes are to a large extent dependent on social, financial, physical and environmental assets at a local level (Jirojwong and Liamputtong, 2009).

Programme needs are typically based on promoting health and preventing disease, whereas the needs of community partners are typically based on addressing local problems. Sometimes these two sets of needs are similar and can be reconciled in the design of the programme. More often, the needs are dissimilar and a compromise has to be found through the design and implementation of the programme. For example, in Auckland, New Zealand, Polynesian people aged 45 years and above have rates for cardiovascular and ischaemic heart disease which are significantly higher (about twice as high) than those in the total population. Polynesian males and females also have higher prevalence rates for diabetes and worse causal-related indicators for obesity, diet, physical exercise and tobacco consumption (Ministry of Health and Ministry of Pacific Island Affairs, 2004). However, public health programmes to promote physical activity, especially amongst Polynesian women, have been unsuccessful because they have failed to recognize the cultural inappropriateness of exercise and other lifestyle activities for women in public places.

A needs assessment approach involves quantitative as well as qualitative methods to determine which needs are a priority, what should be done, what can be done and what can be afforded. In practice, who will participate in the needs assessment is decided through the representation of a few on behalf of the majority, for example, the elected representatives of a community. This is because it is not usually possible for everyone to participate in the needs assessment even when using participatory methods. The diversity of some communities can also create problems with regard to the selection of representatives. Participation can become empty and frustrating for those whose involvement is passive and can sometimes allow those in authority to claim that all sides were considered while only a few benefit.

## Mapping

Mapping is an important stage in needs assessment that includes the identification, ranking and prioritization of the needs and assets of a specific group. There are a number of mapping techniques, mostly based on the principles of collaborative needs assessment, which can be used to engage a large audience. These include whole system planning, values summits, open space and Big Conversation events. While these approaches may be too large, time consuming and expensive for many Practitioners to use, it is worthwhile looking at two examples to illustrate how they work in practice: whole system planning and values summits.

### Whole system planning

Whole system planning is an approach to bring together many diverse sub-group interests to collect information, to understand one another and to build a plan to realign around current and future plans. The event is held in a large space, such as in a community centre or events venue, where people can come together, and follows a process in three parts. The first part focuses on the past to understand the causes of need and if these are still a problem. The next part focuses on the present challenges, strengths and weaknesses. The final part focuses on the future, often beginning with a visioning exercise to determine a desired future state that is then shared, developed and given a local meaning (South et al., 2013).

### Values summits

A values summit brings together a diverse range of people and their perspectives to create a better understanding of how people's differences, social status and cultural expectations can affect their experiences of health and health care. They create a space for patients, the public and citizens to connect with leaders and health professionals and offer a fresh way to talk about, listen to and understand key issues. Values summits typically take two forms: open and closed consultations. Open consultations use informal meetings in, for example, clinical waiting rooms, supermarkets and town squares to ask people about their views on a particular health issue. These events are often a partnership approach with the community services provider, voluntary sector and local authorities all participating in the organization of the event. Closed consultations use anonymous online surveys, questionnaires and individual interviews to gain the views of people on a particular health issue (National Health Service, 2015).

There are a number of other strategies for mapping that can be used within programmes with small, more manageable groups and include community asset mapping (discussed below). The role of the Practitioner is to encourage others to think critically about their own assets, their access to external resources and their ability to make decisions (Rifkin and Pridmore, 2001). Once the needs have been identified, it is the role of the Practitioner to help others to rank them and to move towards decision making and action. When working with local partners who are non-literate, pictures or drawings can be used instead of words to develop a ranked list. The list can then be scored, placing the highest at the top and the lowest at the bottom, to help with prioritization.

## Community asset mapping

Community asset mapping has received considerable attention in, for example, the UK, as a way to foster the 'Big Society agenda'. This concerns moving power away from central government and giving it to local communities and individuals through helping to empower others, changing and opening up public services and promoting social action (South et al., 2013). The steps to successfully undertake a community asset mapping approach include:

▶ The community should identify the assets which they value, as these are likely to have the greatest impact. Individual and community capacities can be considered as assets only in so far as they are valuable to the community.
▶ It is important to consider what the reasons for doing the mapping are and what is hoped to be achieved from it. These considerations are likely to determine the geographic area to be assessed, the size of the sample to be interviewed and the questions to be asked in the mapping exercise.
▶ It is important to consider, early on in the process, how the surveyed assets will be hosted, such as using a database, as this will affect how they may be updated in the future.
▶ It is important to make sure that the final mapping is continually monitored to check whether it is up to date and still useful (NHS North West, 2011).

Mapping can be a time-intensive activity that requires good planning and resources. Experience shows that it is important to involve a variety of stakeholders who can liaise with different segments of local communities. Questionnaires can be an efficient way to systematically collect information on people's personal assets; however, the questions must be able to reach the correct level of detail otherwise the questionnaire will have limited usability. Similarly, local events can be a successful way to undertake asset mapping and offer a context in which to identify specific and individually valued goals (Giuntoli et al., 2012). Practitioners sometimes do not have the skills to use participatory approaches to help others to carry out a needs assessment, and so in Box 3.2 I provide an example of how a semi-participatory approach was used in a school community in Scotland to help students to identify their needs.

### Box 3.2 Needs identification in a school community

Hillhead primary school is in an inner city area in Glasgow, Scotland, with 500 children up to the age of 12 years. The Parents and Teachers Association and children had raised the issue of accidents both inside and outside the school environment. The Practitioners wanted to find out from the children about their perspectives of school safety and how they would like to make it a safer environment as part of the design of a public health intervention. The younger children were encouraged to describe the safe and unsafe areas of the school and on their journey to and from the school by using a

*(Continued)*

drawing. The older children were shown epidemiological data in a visual format using bar charts, pie charts and graphs of school and road accidents in the Glasgow area. These children were asked what they thought this information meant: why did more accidents happen to boys, why did they happened at certain times of the day and in certain places? The children provided very thoughtful answers, even raising the issue of reporting bias, and this provided a different perspective to the Practitioners. The children were asked for their ideas on how to redesign the school playground and on any new rules that they would like to introduce to help make their school a safer place. The children's suggestions included painting the edges of stairs, removing spikes from railings, creating a quiet area of the playground with benches where children could rest away from the rough and tumble of the playground, and staggering playtimes to allow the younger children to play and to avoid older children. The Practitioner could then use the ideas put forward by the participants as part of a planning process for community actions, supported by an outside agency (Roberts, 1998).

In Box 3.3 I provide the example of the 'story with a gap', a simple visual technique to enable people to analyse important needs shared by their community and then to develop strategies to address them.

### Box 3.3 Analysing community needs: The story with a gap

The 'story with a gap' is a tool that is used to stimulate discussion about the causes of and the solutions to priority needs at the community level. The technique begins when each group is given two large pictures. One picture shows the before situation of a community priority, for example, a road traffic accident. The group is asked to develop a story about their community and the issues that they have encountered due to traffic in their area. The participants are encouraged to make the story realistic by including the names of places and people. The second picture shows the after situation, for example, slow-moving traffic regulated by traffic lights or speed bumps. The group is asked to develop a story which explains how this improvement has occurred. The stories that they develop will 'fill the gap' between the two pictures. The group members are asked to recount their story and the content is discussed to identify possible pathways to the solutions. The tool allows participants to generate ideas about how the community can organize itself to find solutions which they feel have a high priority. The Practitioner facilitates this process of discovery and is part of building specific skills necessary for community capacity (Srinivasan, 1993).

## Parallel-tracking empowerment

A major challenge in public health is how to accommodate bottom-up needs within top-down programmes. To achieve this goal the process of empowerment can be better viewed as a 'parallel track' running alongside the main public health programme track.

The tensions, rather than being conventionally viewed as a top-down versus bottom-up tension, can then occur at each stage of the programme cycle, making their resolution practicable. Parallel-tracking helps to move our professional thinking on from a simple bottom-up/top-down dichotomy. Through parallel-tracking, the financial, material, human and other resources can be systematically made available in a more empowering way through the delivery of the programme.

In parallel-tracking the purpose of the programme itself changes to become a pathway through which bottom-up needs are intentionally formalized, rather than being viewed as a secondary benefit. The programming issue at stake is how both the public health track and the empowerment track become linked during the progressive stages of the programme cycle, namely: objective setting; the strategic approach; management and implementation; and evaluation.

The parallel-track is illustrated in Figure 3.1, which shows each of the different stages of the cycle in a maternal and newborn health programme.

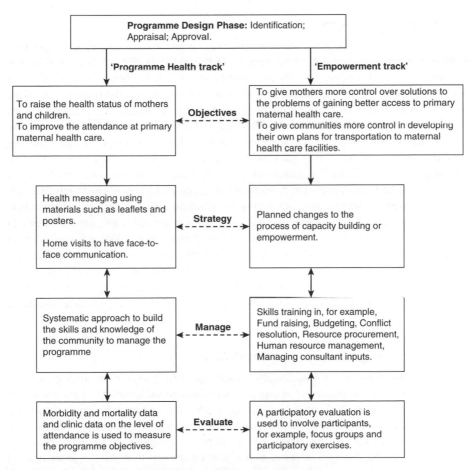

**Figure 3.1**  Parallel-tracking maternal and newborn health programmes

## Parallel-tracking in a maternal and newborn health programme

### Setting programme objectives

Objective setting within conventional top-down programming is usually centred on dis-ease prevention, a reduction in morbidity and mortality and lifestyle management, such as a change in specific health-related behaviours. The issue is how to give empowerment objectives an equal priority with the disease prevention objectives and to reflect this in the parallel-track. The Practitioner must first ascertain from the participants what are their needs are, as discussed earlier, and this information is then used to set the empower-ment objectives, which have to be achievable and measurable. For example, in maternal and newborn health these might include programme objectives to raise the health status of mothers and children and to improve attendance at primary maternal health care centres. Empowerment objectives might include giving mothers more control over solu-tions to gain better access to primary maternal health care and to give communities more control in developing their own plans for the transportation of pregnant women to health care centres.

### Develop the strategic approach

It is important that the approach used by the programme is paralleled by strategies that build community capacity and empowerment. In this example, the objectives are to raise the health status of mothers and children and to improve the attendance of mothers at primary maternal health care facilities. To achieve these objectives the programme might typically employ communication and behaviour change strategies; for example, health education materials, talks by nurses to mothers and visits to households to discuss the importance of attending primary maternal health facilities. Strategies for strengthening the empowerment of mothers to gain more control in regard to primary maternal health care might include building the capacity of women's groups to address, for example, better transportation services or collective fund raising to support the cost of childbirth and care. There is also strong evidence that community mobilization with women's groups has a wide range of benefits, such as cost-effectiveness, reductions in mortality and improvements in the health of newborn infants, children and mothers (Rosato et al., 2008). It is important to set short-term performance goals, for example, the formation of a women's group, because these achievable successes can help to motivate people towards longer-term objectives. The progress should be periodically reviewed to reflect on success and failures to build capacity and this can be achieved through using, for example, the domains approach as discussed in Chapter 9.

### Programme management and implementation

The management process is traditionally concerned with planning, organizing, leading and controlling the utilization of resources, both human and material, to achieve the programme objectives (O'Connor and Parker, 1995). The person who controls, or has power-over, this process determines the direction and sometimes the success of achieving the objectives. In more general terms management is concerned with effectiveness, the extent to which objectives are achieved, and efficiency, the way in which the objectives are achieved compared to other means (Ewles and Simnett, 2003). The role of the Practitioner is to be sympathetic to help make the management process an empowering experience for the participants through involvement in activities such as reporting, budgeting and evaluation. In order for programme participants to have the confidence to undertake more responsibilities they may have to acquire specific skills.

Table 3.2 provides a list of relevant skills training for community members that can be systematically incorporated by the Practitioner as part of a management plan of the programme.

**Table 3.2** Developing skills in public health planning and management

| Programme phase | Skills training |
| --- | --- |
| Design | ▶ Analysis of epidemiological data.<br>▶ Identification of community needs.<br>▶ Appraisal of programme design. |
| Objective setting | ▶ Writing SMART objectives.<br>▶ Framework development. |
| Strategic approach | ▶ Strategies to empower individuals, groups and communities.<br>▶ Public health models and theories.<br>▶ Interpersonal communication.<br>▶ Workshop facilitation.<br>▶ Conducting effective group meetings and public presentation. |
| Programme management and implementation | ▶ Fund raising.<br>▶ Budgeting.<br>▶ Conflict resolution.<br>▶ Resource procurement.<br>▶ Human resource management. |
| Evaluation | ▶ Participatory rural appraisal techniques.<br>▶ Qualitative research methods.<br>▶ Quantitative research methods. |

Laverack (2007, p. 57).

## Evaluation of the programme

The final stage in the programme cycle is normally an evaluation of the outcomes, often set against the objectives, although mid-term evaluations and monitoring can also be carried out. In parallel-tracking the aim is that both the programme and empowerment objectives are evaluated. Empowerment outcomes may not occur until after the time frame of the programme, normally two to five years. Thus, the evaluation of community empowerment within a programme context can be more appropriately assessed as a process as well as specific outcomes. Programme success in terms of empowerment is best judged in terms of how the participants, through a self-assessment, experience improvements in their lives and health. The evaluation therefore needs to employ participatory methods that draw upon the experiences and knowledge of the programme participants. There is also the need to be systematic in the way in which we evaluate community empowerment, how we compare the information collected over time, between respondents and between communities within the same programme and how we present and interpret this information. Later I describe the measurement and visual representation of community empowerment and discuss how this information can be used to quickly interpret the strengths and weaknesses of a community.

Next, Chapter 4 addresses how public health practitioners can help individuals to become empowered through a greater sense of autonomy, by overcoming powerlessness and by becoming more effective communicators, learning to listen and developing a dialogue.

# 4

# HELPING INDIVIDUALS TO BECOME EMPOWERED

Helping individuals to become empowered begins by building power-from-within and helping others to participate in groups that share their interests. It is collective rather than individual empowerment that eventually brings about the broader social and political changes that can improve people's lives and health. However, the ability of the individual to overcome powerlessness, to improve their personal competencies and to build their power-from-within is crucial to gaining a greater collective influence.

## Autonomy

Autonomy refers to the capacity to be self-governing, to make the decisions that will influence one's life and health. It is linked to what it is to be a person, to be able to choose freely and to be able to formulate how one wants to live one's life (Kant et al., 1997). A respect for the autonomy of the individual and for the conditions in people's lives that support such autonomy is core to an ethical and empowering approach to public health.

Autonomy and empowerment are closely connected as both relate to having the freedom and opportunities in our lives to be able to make the right choices for ourselves. The difference between delivering an empowering approach in contrast to delivering a behaviour change approach is also closely related to autonomy in public health programmes. If, for example, the programme gives the Practitioner more authority in setting the agenda, it is less likely to be empowering for others. If it facilitates a process of needs assessment, planning and capacity building, it has a much better chance of being empowering. In a professional context the key question is: Do I want to help to empower people or to simply change their behaviour? Both approaches aim to achieve improvements in health; however, the advantage of empowerment is that it also strengthens autonomy and control in achieving healthier and more sustainable lives. Behaviour changes do sometimes lead to more autonomy and control, but, if they do, this is usually as a secondary outcome, for example, a feeling of greater self-esteem following smoking cessation. Public health programmes should not simply aim to change behaviour but should also aim for the attainment of more autonomous choice at an individual level (Laverack, 2015).

It is the Practitioner, or their agency, that usually provides the initial direction and enthusiasm for the programme. This is contradictory to an empowering approach in which the issue to be addressed should involve the beneficiaries of the programme. However, some clients may not want to have more control in their lives, especially if they have lived under powerless circumstances and feel that they do not have the right or do not possess the ability to empower themselves. For other people, health is secondary to their personal goals and they may be willing to risk their well-being by pursuing an unhealthy lifestyle. What must be remembered is that power cannot be given. People must gain it for themselves. The right to be empowered rests with the individual and the role of the Practitioner is to facilitate and enable others to take greater responsibility over their lives. Some people may fear the regret of making a misjudgement and therefore are willing to delegate control to another person in whom they have trust. Others, such as the very young, the very old or people with an addiction, may not have the ability to sufficiently organize themselves. Public health practice may then intervene; for example, through policy and legislation to protect population health, to reduce vehicle speed limits to protect drivers and pedestrians, and to restrict the sale of alcohol and tobacco to children (Baum, 2008).

## Overcoming powerlessness

As discussed in Chapter 2, powerlessness is the absence of power, whether imagined or real, and is a personal concept with the expectancy that the behaviour of an individual or group cannot determine the outcomes they seek (Kieffer, 1984). Powerlessness is a barrier to gaining control in one's life and is something that both Practitioners and their clients can experience. For Practitioners this might mean the actions of an authorative manager controlling the decisions they make; for example, micro-managing the work of the ward nurses in a hospital. For a client this might mean a Practitioner showing indifference about their needs or being excluded from decisions about their health care. It is important that the Practitioner is able to recognize their own position of powerlessness, because, as I discuss in Chapter 2, before they can help to empower others they must first empower themselves. The exercise in Box 4.1 allows Practitioners to begin to think critically, to discuss and to support one another in regard to their own positions of powerlessness in a work setting.

---

**Box 4.1 Examining positions of professional powerlessness**

This exercise can be carried out in small groups or on an individual basis. The Practitioners are asked to produce a description (written or pictorial) of themselves in a position where the Director of Nursing (or another person in authority to them) has power-over them in their work setting. The Practitioners are then asked:

- How do you feel in this situation?
- What is the basis for your sense of powerlessness?
- How can you change the situation to make yourselves feel more comfortable?
- What simple strategies could your apply to empower yourselves?

The Practitioners are encouraged to discuss their answers with the whole group and the facilitator develops a discussion around some of the key issues raised. The facilitator can write the main points and strategies onto a board so that all the Practitioners can see the outcome of the discussion.

---

In Box 4.2 I provide another exercise on weaning practices to help Practitioners to understand how they can use their power to help to empower others. In many countries women do not make decisions in isolation from the context of their lives and this involves asking other family members for advice. In this example, Heidi, a young mother, has been advised by a nurse to exclusively breastfeed her child until it is six months old. The nurse has explained the nutritional, health protective and child-spacing benefits of breastfeeding, as well as showing Heidi how to initiate skin contact and to hold her child to encourage her to feed and bond with the mother. However, Heidi's mother is encouraging her to wean the baby at three months by feeding it porridge. This is Heidi's first child and she is very anxious about giving her baby the best start in life but feels under considerable family pressure to wean her child too early. Heidi feels powerless, depressed and anxious about the safety of her child and asks another nurse Practitioner to help with this decision making process.

---

### Box 4.2 Powerlessness and weaning practices

What should the nurse do to help empower Heidi?

After discussing the example of Heidi in groups, the participants are asked to share their ideas on how to help Heidi, based on the introduction to the concepts of power and empowerment. These ideas can be written on a whiteboard or large sheet of paper to display them to other participants.

**Possible discussion points**

1. The nurse Practitioner uses her authority and professional status to lend credibility to Heidi's concerns. 2. Mentoring the woman to identify her own power bases (social support, family, friends) to strengthen her power-from-within. 3. Using her power-over (status, authority), the nurse Practitioner can advocate to the head of the family ('I'll do this, but only if you'll consider how to learn to do it yourselves...'); the nurse Practitioner exercises her control with the intent of increasing the power-from-within of Heidi and her family.

---

To build power-from-within, the Practitioner can use strategies to increase feelings of value and a sense of control in their clients. While the ability of the Practitioner to be an effective communicator can help the way in which people feel about themselves, individuals become more powerful through their own sense of worth. There are a number of strategies that can help individuals to build their power-from-within, but it would be unrealistic to expect Practitioners to use them all. I therefore select some low-cost and effective strategies that can be used as part of everyday work: Practitioners as more effective communicators; harm reduction; and moral suasion.

## Practitioners as more effective communicators

Practitioners often use health communication in their everyday work to impart information to their clients, to advocate on behalf of their clients or to mediate between conflicting interest groups. Health communication is the exchange of information in regard to health issues to raise awareness and to develop a dialogue with people. The communication can be individually focused on a one-to-one (Practitioner-to-client) basis, for example, a doctor talking to a patient in his/her surgery. The communication can also be used to reach a larger audience, for example, a group discussion that is used to develop a dialogue between a nurse and a group of mothers waiting at a well-baby clinic. Communication can help individuals to gain more control over their lives by providing specific information that allows them to make an informed choice, for example, about the benefits of breastfeeding or immunization. Communication can also help individuals to increase their understanding about the underlying causes of their powerlessness, for example, the reasons they receive a lower income than their colleagues.

## Learning to listen

Listening is integral to becoming a more effective communicator: the Practitioner needs to focus on what the individual is saying and to help them to express their feelings or to give an opinion on a specific need. When giving advice, the Practitioner is exerting their expert and legitimate power to persuade the client into actually accepting a subservient role in the relationship. The relationship grants the Practitioner the right to prescribe advice, while the client accepts an obligation to comply with the advice. This can relate to a range of different types of information. The Practitioner may also use their power-over in a form of dominance to control the choice of their client. This is sometimes a necessary communication style when, for example, giving a precise instruction, such as the self-treatment of a wound by the patient, to ensure compliance. Obtaining and giving feedback enables the Practitioner to clarify what the client needs, that they have understood previous communication or have retained skills. This may mean obtaining feedback based on specific information using closed questions that require short factual (yes/no) answers or based on a more open form of questioning to allow a fuller response. Giving feedback is important for the achievement of effective communication and, in particular, positive feedback that can reinforce the strengths of the client's knowledge or their skill level. To facilitate the listening process the Practitioner can use people-centred approaches, such as the patient-centred clinical method (see Chapter 5) that applies the principles of empowerment in a Practitioner–client relationship.

A critical variable in communication approaches is the process of problem solving and this has been used, for example, in diabetes self-management. One systematic review of studies reporting problem-solving interventions for diabetes self-management found that 36% of adult interventions and 42% of children/adolescent interventions had demonstrated a significant improvement in diabetes, while psychosocial outcomes had been even more promising (Fitzpatrick et al., 2013).

## An exercise to help Practitioners become more effective communicators

The following is a simple exercise that helps Practitioners to think carefully about how they can communicate with their clients, in this case in regard to the preparation for the home delivery of a newborn child (World Health Organization, 2007a). In this exercise the participants are divided into groups of three people. Each group is asked to designate someone who will be the 'Practitioner', someone who will be the 'mother' and someone who will be an impartial 'observer'. The role of the 'observer' is to watch the interaction between the 'Practitioner' and the 'mother' without making any comments on their conversation.

The 'observer' uses table 4.1 to record the level of interaction and communication between the 'Practitioner' and the 'mother'. The 'Practitioner' and the 'mother' are given table 4.2 and asked to carefully consider the circumstances of planning for the birth of the mother's child. They are not told how to do this by the facilitator. The mode of interaction is decided upon by both participants and this automatically sets up a power dynamic between the 'Practitioner' and 'mother'. This dynamic will vary depending on the power-from-within and power-over of the two people. The 'Practitioner' and 'mother' are to sit together to complete the actions identified to resolve the concern and place them in some order of priority. The first suggested action has been provided in Table 4.2 to encourage discussion.

After the exercise has finished, the participants discuss their experiences as the 'Practitioner', the 'mother' and the 'observer' in a plenary session. The facilitator can ask, for example:

1  What did they feel about the level of one-to-one communication?
2  Did the Practitioner use empowering language?
3  Did the Practitioner listen to the mother?
4  Did the Practitioner facilitate the mother to help her to make her own decisions?

Table 4.3 provides an example of some potential actions that can be developed by the mother to plan for a delivery and is also shared with the participants in the plenary session after the exercise.

**Table 4.1**   Communication skills checklist

| Did the 'Practitioner' ...? | Yes | No | Comments from observer |
|---|---|---|---|
| Introduce themselves to the mother | | | |
| Use the mother's name | | | |
| Greet the mother | | | |
| Explain their role and purpose | | | |
| Ensure that the mother was comfortable | | | |
| Establish and maintain eye contact | | | |
| Listen to what the mother was saying | | | |
| Use open-ended questions | | | |
| Inform the mother that information would be recorded | | | |
| Maintain interest in what the mother was saying during note taking | | | |
| Identify and respond to verbal and non-verbal cues | | | |
| Give appropriate and accurate advice | | | |
| Provide a summary of what was said and agreed | | | |
| Obtain feedback from the mother | | | |
| Give a pleasant thank you and farewell | | | |

Adapted from Lloyd and Bor (2004, p. 190)

Table 4.2

| Column 1.<br>Priority concern expressed by the mother. | Column 2.<br>Actions identified to resolve this concern. |
|---|---|
| Do not have a plan for the birth of their child? (Where will the birth take place? By whom? How will you get there?) | Develop a birth plan with clear roles and responsibilities and shared decision making for a husband, wife and family. |

Table 4.3

| Column 1.<br>Priority concern expressed by the mother. | Column 2.<br>Actions identified to resolve this concern. |
|---|---|
| Do not have a plan for the birth of their child? (Where will the birth take place? By whom? How will you get there?) | Develop a birth plan with clear roles and responsibilities and shared decision making for man, wife and family.<br><br>Identify who will take the mother to the place of delivery and who will stay with her during labour.<br><br>Access to information about what will happen during labour, the danger signs leading up to giving birth and postnatal self-care.<br><br>Have adequate supplies for the birth (new blade in clean cover, clean thread, at least five cloths, washed and dried in the sun, change of clothes, food and drink). |

World Health Organization (2007a).

An assessment of communication involving listening, giving advice and obtaining and providing feedback can be an important part of the learning process for Practitioners. The communication skills checklist provided in table 4.1 can be used by trainers in role-play or work practice sessions. The Practitioner is observed by the trainer, or by another participant, who completes each section of the checklist and then provides feedback. The identified strengths of interpersonal communication and the areas that need further work are then discussed to improve the communication ability of the Practitioner.

## One-to-one communication

One-to-one communication is important, because this allows a dialogue to develop between the client and the Practitioner. The dialogue is often based on a sharing of knowledge and experiences in a two-way communication that is necessary to help individuals to better retain information, to clarify personal issues and to develop skills. Verbal communication is a common method of relaying information between the Practitioner and the client. Situations where one-to-one communication takes place include providing health advice to an individual and counselling someone on a sensitive issue, such as the result of a medical test.

It is important to emphasize that the choice of the communication style is usually at the discretion of the Practitioner, who decides, based on the circumstances and the type of client, what is most appropriate. For example, using a controlling approach, such as a direct instruction to make the client take a prescribed medication, might be seen as an unethical imposition of the Practitioner's values. This can be reinforced through non-verbal communication, for example, body language, posture and facial expressions. Whenever possible the Practitioner should consider a communication style that is non-controlling, such as the GATHER approach outlined in Box 4.3.

---

**Box 4.3 The GATHER approach in one-to-one communication**

G   Greet the clients, make them feel comfortable, show respect, trust and empathy.

A   Ask them about their problem: help them to talk about their problems and needs, listen to them and encourage their feedback.

T   Tell them any relevant information: provide technical information about their health issue, use simple language and focus on the important points.

H   Help them to make decisions: by exploring the options to their particular circumstances and by developing a realistic action plan.

E   Explain any misunderstandings: ask questions and clarify any issues raised.

R   Return to follow up on them: revisit, make a reappointment or refer the clients to another practitioner to ensure that the issues were understood and acted upon. Obtain and give feedback. (Adapted from Walley et al., 2001, p. 163)

---

Counselling is a form of one-to-one communication and refers to any interaction where someone seeks to explore, understand or resolve a problem or a troubling personal aspect of their life. Counselling occurs broadly when a person consults someone else in regard to a problem, conflict or dilemma that is preventing them from living their lives in a way that they would wish to do so (McLeod and McLeod, 2011). Essentially, counselling can involve people working in any kind of helping, managing or facilitative role such as social work. Counselling can be done with a single person or with couples or a small group and may be delivered through methods such as one-to-one communication, group work (Dryden and Feltham, 1993), interpersonal communication, interviewing and shared decision making. Listening is also a key skill in counselling and in the everyday work of health professionals, and Box 4.4 provides three quick exercises that can be used to help Practitioners and their clients to better understand the importance of listening in the process of communication.

---

**Box 4.4 Three short exercises to help Practitioners and their clients to listen**

Exercise 1. Pair up participants and have one person discuss a health issue such as the importance of regular exercise, while the other person is instructed to ignore them. Discuss the frustration that can come with not feeling heard or being acknowledged, and review body language and verbal remarks that a good listener should practise.

Exercise 2. One participant discusses a health condition, for example, a sprained ankle, giving only subtle hints as to the specific nature of the condition to the listener.

*(Continued)*

The listener will have to pick up on these subtleties and at the end recommend suitable advice for the speaker about treatment or care. The two participants will then discuss the ways that people can more actively communicate and listen to what others are saying.

Exercise 3. The group of participants should stand in a circle. One person begins the game by whispering a message to the person next to them. This message (for example, 'Think before you act; keep your hands and feet clear.') should be prepared beforehand, by the facilitator, who is the only person who knows the exact wording. The person who receives the message should then whisper it to the person next to them, moving clockwise around the circle. When it reaches the final person in the group they should say the message aloud. The first person will read the message they were given, and participants can then see how different the two messages are, as it is unlikely that the message has not been altered during the process of communication and listening. The group can discuss the principles of good listening.

## Harm reduction

Harm reduction is a pragmatic approach that can directly help individuals to reduce the harmful consequences of high-risk behaviours by incorporating strategies that cover safer use, managed use and abstinence. High-risk behaviours that have been included in harm reduction interventions are needle exchange, opioid substitution therapy, substance use prevention for adolescents, smoking cessation, homelessness and sex work (Ritter and Cameron, 2006). The principles of harm reduction are often rooted in the recognition that risky behaviours have always been and always will be a part of society. The primary goal of harm reduction is to work with individuals on their terms in their context and not to condemn their behaviours but to minimize the harmful effects of a given behaviour. Unlike the moral approach, which tends to enhance the user's shame, guilt and feelings of stigma, the harm reduction approach is based on acceptance and the willingness of the provider to collaborate with clients in the course of reducing harmful consequences (Marlatt and Witkiewitz, 2010). The term 'harm minimization' is sometimes used interchangeably with 'harm reduction'. However, the term harm minimization is intended to reflect an overall goal of policies to minimize harm (Weatherburn, 2009).

One harm reduction intervention used brief motivational interviews to reduce alcohol-related consequences among adolescents (aged 18–19 years) treated in an emergency room following an alcohol-related event. An assessment of their condition and future risk of harm and the motivational interviews were conducted in the emergency room during or after the patient's treatment. Follow-up assessments showed that patients who received the motivational interviews had a significantly lower incidence of drinking and driving, traffic violations, alcohol-related injuries and alcohol-related problems than patients who only received the standard care in the emergency room (Monti et al., 1999).

There is opposition to harm reduction strategies from some Practitioners who want to eliminate high-risk behaviours by enforcing abstinence-only policies. This is despite the widespread evidence that harm reduction programmes can be effective and cost-efficient, for example, in slowing down the spread of HIV and other communicable diseases, overdose prevention programmes and in emergency room screening and workplace substance use prevention programmes (Marlatt and Witkiewitz, 2010).

In practice, harm reduction is most viable as an approach in public health when it is used in combination with other strategies, such as peer education, to manage high-risk behaviours. Peer education is an approach in which people are supported to promote health-enhancing change among their peers. Rather than health professionals educating members of the public, lay persons are felt to be in the best position to encourage each other to adopt healthy behaviours. Peer education has become very popular in the field of HIV prevention, especially involving young people, sex workers, men who have sex with men and intravenous drug users. Peer education is also associated with efforts to prevent tobacco, drug or alcohol use among young people, teenage pregnancy and homelessness (UNAIDS, 1999).

## Moral suasion

Moral suasion is the act of trying to use moral principles to influence individuals to change their practices, beliefs and actions (Laverack, 2014, p. 132). Moral suasion is a form of persuasion based on moral reasoning to change people's beliefs and behaviours. Persuasion is a process aimed at changing a person's (or a group's) attitude, belief or behaviour towards some event or idea by using methods of communication including spoken words to convey information, feelings or reasoning. Persuasion can also be interpreted as using one's personal or positional resources to gain leverage to change people's behaviours or attitudes (Seiter and Gass, 2010).

The temperance movement, for example, used a strategy of moral suasion to oppose the drinking of spirits and beer to the point of total abstinence in the UK in the nineteenth century. The strategy concentrated on the establishment of a mass movement of mostly men to take a 'pledge' to cease the use of alcohol. The movement offered support through a set of self-help groups and worked across the classes in society advocating for a sober workforce as well as for 'teetotallers' (total abstinence) everywhere (Berridge, 2007). A similar approach was used in regard to foot-binding, which was painful and dangerous and afflicted Chinese women for a millennium. And yet this practice ended, for the most part, in a single generation. The natural-foot movement was championed by liberal modernizers and women's rights advocates and developed in the years of change culminating in the Revolution of 1911. Reform and urban economic development were part of modernization and mass migration from the countryside. This consequently provided alternative opportunities of support for women, strengthening their financial independence and bargaining power. The natural-foot movement used moral suasion by forming alliances, called 'pledge associations', of parents who promised not to foot-bind their daughters nor let their sons marry foot-bound women (Mackie, 1996) as moral principles for the basis of individual behaviour change. An important element in the process of mobilizing individuals in the fight against female genital mutilation (FGM) has also used moral suasion. Public statements or declarations can take different forms, including signing a statement, alternative rites of passage celebrations and multi-village gatherings. When public statements are made, this suggests that a sufficient number of individuals have decided, on moral grounds, not to have their children cut and to abandon FGM, which can further promote broad-scale abandonment. The public statements can mark a final decision to abandon FGM or are a milestone that signifies readiness for change and indicates that further support is needed to sustain and accelerate the process (Johansen et al., 2013).

Next, Chapter 5 addresses the contemporary field of patient empowerment, the importance of the professional–patient relationship and discusses approaches to achieve patient self-management. Chapter 5 also discusses the role that advocacy, networks and involvement action groups can play in the broader empowerment of patients.

# 5

# PATIENT EMPOWERMENT

## Introduction

Historically, patient empowerment has derived from two different points of view based on the professional–patient power relationship. One is that compliance with Practitioner instructions is critical to good health. The other is that the health of individuals improves not merely by complying with instructions but also when the patient becomes actively involved in decisions about his/her own health. The first view is one that is embedded in the bio-medical interpretation of health, while the second is embedded in its socio-economic interpretation. Health professionals have traditionally controlled the management of disease, thus relieving patients of responsibility, but patient empowerment is increasingly recognized as being important, especially in illnesses that require both drug compliance and a life-style change, for example, in the case of diabetes (Rifkin, 2006). There has also been a shift in which patients want, even demand, to be more involved in health decision making. A review of 115 patient participation studies found that the majority of respondents preferred to participate in medical decision making in only 50% of studies prior to 2000 compared to 71% of studies after 2000 (Chewning et al., 2012). Practitioners now have to consider more carefully how they can involve patients within the health systems that they work in and within the interpretation of health that they use.

The role of education in patient empowerment is not to coerce people into following specific instructions but to enable them to increase their self-reliance and to make autonomous choices. Patient education increasingly uses decision making aids that assist patients in choosing the treatment and health care options that most closely align with their values and preferences. These aids, for example, interactive media, may also help to increase patients' trust and facilitate the shared professional–patient decision making process (van Til et al., 2010). For example, one survey of 1700 patients in the UK accessing a health information website showed a high patient demand for online health services, such as booking GP (General Practitioner) appointments and ordering repeat medication. Almost half of the respondents (47%) were aged over 55, indicating that demand for internet-based health services is not limited to younger patients and that over three-quarters of respondents (78%) were female (Patient UK, 2012). A major barrier to patient education is the assumption by some Practitioners that they play a dominant role and they may resist changes for a more equal partnership with their clients and a broader understanding of health (Rifkin, 2006).

## What is patient empowerment?

Patient empowerment enables people to take control of their health, well-being and disease management and to participate in decisions affecting their care. Patient empowerment involves respecting patients' rights, and giving people a 'voice' so that they can collectively participate in making health systems more user friendly and health information more accessible (Lancet, 2012).

Patient empowerment is different to the traditional approach to care that tends to ignore personal preferences and creates a dependency on the Practitioner and on health systems. The professional relationship is traditionally paternalistic and unequal, where the expertise is considered to belong to the person with the most control, the Practitioner. Patient empowerment can therefore sometimes be in conflict with the ideology of the traditional health professional–patient relationship. Patient empowerment is unlikely to be successful unless Practitioners understand a fundamental principle: before they can empower others they must first be empowered themselves and understand the sources of their own power. To build a more empowering practice the constraints of working in institutional and bureaucratic settings, which do not necessarily share an ideology of empowerment, must be redressed (see Chapter 1). This has been argued in the context of a nursing profession that can only become empowered when individual nurses themselves have more control in hospital settings (Kendall, 1998). Nurses work to enable patients to take more control in decision making over their health, promote independence, provide information and address patient needs. In practice, this translates into acts of everyday care, such as making sure patients have their call bell within reach, providing information about future care options and working quietly at night to allow patients to sleep (Faulkner, 2001).

There is no universally accepted measure of patient empowerment, although different tools have used similar dimensions based on individual decision making, control, self-efficacy and the self-management of chronic disease. Patient-reported outcome measures include self-reporting questionnaires, including Patient Enablement Instruments, Patient Activation Measures and Diabetes Empowerment Scales. In the USA, self-completion questionnaires have been used to capture aspects of patient satisfaction, such as the degree of involvement in decision making about their care. But approaches based on patient satisfaction do not capture true outcomes of empowerment or of the effectiveness of a health care intervention. Models for the measurement of patient empowerment must include a consensus between patients, clinicians and policy makers about the content and boundaries of the construct before implementation. The measurement should also include indicators for process, outcome and impact as well as for individual and collective action (McAllister et al., 2012).

## The professional–patient power relationship

The delicate balance at the professional–patient level can be illustrated in the doctor–patient relationship. The doctor (after an examination) tells the patient what their medical problem is and prescribes a treatment for it. The patient voluntarily surrenders to the medical (expert) power of the doctor and the phrase 'Doctor knows best' epitomizes this situation. The doctor has control over the knowledge even though this concerns the patient's own body. The attributes of health are viewed as an individual case history and the diagnosis is made on the basis of the medical approach (the presence or absence of disease or illness) that serves to protect the expert power held by the doctor. However, in the health system, the power-over relationship does not stop at diagnosis because the doctor often also controls the admission and discharge, choice of treatment, referral and care of the patient (Laverack, 2007). One example of this is a consultation between a health professional and a pregnant woman. The Practitioner began the discussion using 'lay' terms to describe the complications associated with her condition but quickly switched to a technical-rational language when her advice was challenged by the patient. The patient was then coerced into complying with the Practitioner because she suddenly felt uncertain and lacking in knowledge. The patient had been disempowered by the Practitioner, who said that she was unaware of the switch to a technical, power-over use of language (Scrambler, 1987). This type of an approach can contribute to a sense of powerlessness by emphasizing a lack of access to knowledge and the expert power of the other person who is in control, the Practitioner.

A more equal relationship would be one in which the Practitioner uses their knowledge to allow the patient to make informed decisions about their treatment and recovery. In effect, the patient is placed at the centre of the issue, requiring the Practitioner to gain as much information as possible from their experience rather than what the Practitioner should achieve in the consultation. In one study, for example, a videotaped nurse–patient health counselling session was conducted in a hospital, and this was found to improve the professional–patient working relationship. The investigator separately interviewed the nurse and the patient after the interaction in which the nurse encouraged the patient to speak out, tactfully assessed the patient's concerns and knowledge of impending surgery, listened to feedback and built a positive vision of the future for the patient. The nurse also paid particular attention to the different forms of technical language that she used in the discussion to enable the patient to gain more self-confidence (Kettunen et al., 2001). Box 5.1 provides the outline of a systematic method, the patient-centred clinical method, which applies the principles of empowerment in the professional–patient relationship.

## Box 5.1 The patient-centred clinical method

1 The illness and the patient's experience of being ill are explored at the same time.
2 Understanding the person as a whole places the illness into context by considering how the illness affects the person, how the person interacts with their immediate environment and how the wider environment influences this interaction.
3 The patient and professional reach a mutual understanding of the nature of the illness, its causes and the goals for its management, and who is responsible for what.
4 The desirability and applicability of undertaking broader health promoting tasks; for example, providing the patient with information or skills about how they can dress their own wound at home.
5 Gaining a better understanding of the patient–professional relationship in order to enhance it; for example, placing a value on the contribution being made by both sides and forming a 'partnership' to address the illness rather than a traditional paternalistic approach.
6 Making a realistic assessment of what can be done to help the patient given constraints in knowledge, time and skill level. (Stewart et al., 2003)

## Chronic disease management

Chronic disease management is not intended as a substitute for professional acute care, but by learning to self-manage patients with chronic diseases are more likely to remain integrated in society and the workforce. Chronic disease self-management can help people to gain confidence and acquire the skills to recognize warning symptoms, take medication and decide about the treatment that is best suited to them (Lancet, 2012). Giving the patient more control over decisions that influence their health, well-being and recovery can occur as part of home-based treatment, care for the dying (palliative care) and chronic conditions. Box 5.2 provides an example of how giving a patient more control over decisions related to home-based care can yield real benefits.

---

### Box 5.2 Home-based care and patient empowerment

Giving the patient more control over decisions can have real benefits, as demonstrated in one study (Bassett and Prapavessis, 2007) on physical therapy for ankle sprains. The study showed that the home-based groups had similar outcome scores for post-treatment ankle function, adherence and motivation to a standard physical therapy intervention. However, the home-based group had significantly better attendance at clinic appointments and a better physical therapy completion rate. Patients were helped to set goals and to develop personal action plans to complete the therapy as well as education and skills training on the treatment, such as strapping techniques. The patients had more control and were better informed about their recovery, and this sharing of the power (knowledge, skills) by the Practitioner was a form of power-with, which led to a viable home-based option for the patients. Self-care can be a complicated issue that is not appropriate for all situations or people but under the right conditions, as this study showed, can offer the Practitioner the opportunity to work in a more empowering way.

---

Nevertheless, self-care can be a complicated issue that is not appropriate for all situations or for all patients, and the importance of arranging for patients to choose the nature or timing of treatment, or teaching them 'coping skills' in groups, has shown variable results (Salmon and Hall, 2004).

## Fostering an empowering professional–patient relationship

Fostering an empowering professional–patient relationship describes a process in which power-over is deliberately used by the Practitioner to increase the power-from-within of the patient. This is the transformative use of power-with as described in Chapter 2. The qualities of an empowering relationship include a non-coercive dialogue between the Practitioner and the patient in the identification of problems and solutions. The key attributes of the Practitioner in an empowering role are as an enabler, facilitator, helper and guide to support their patients to facilitate change in their health through their own actions. However, not all Practitioners can apply an empowering approach to their everyday work; for example, those involved in enforcement, licensing and legal proceedings will have fewer opportunities to empower others than those working in an advisory role, as a communicator, a listener or helping people to become more critically aware (Chapter 6).

A combination of approaches is often more effective in helping to empower patients; for example, a review of the literature to examine how empowerment can be effectively used in pain management for patients with cancer identified strategies to promote self-efficacy, active participation, increasing abilities and the control over events in a person's life. However, most strategies focused on pain treatment either induced by the professional or with the active involvement of the patient and not on a combination of both approaches. The review recommended focusing on pain treatment given by the professional, with the active involvement of the patient, and on the interaction of both the professional and the patient in decision making (Boveldt et al., 2014).

An empowering professional–patient relationship involves a discourse, ideology and language that are crucial in linking the individual with their social and political context. The language that we choose to use as professionals can therefore have a significant influence upon the people with whom we work, and it is the power of language in public health that I next discuss.

## The power of language

Language exerts considerable force in our world constructions in both our professional as well as our social contexts (Seidman and Wagner, 1992). In particular, the way in which 'to empower', the central action in an empowering public health practice, has been interpreted is critical. Labonté (1994, p. 255) discusses the transitive and intransitive meanings of the verb 'to empower'. The transitive (direct) meaning is to 'bestow power on others, an enabling act, sharing some of the power we hold over others'. Empowerment is cast as a relationship between the stakeholders of a programme, those with power-over and those without power. Empowerment becomes a dynamic in which this relationship continually shifts towards a more empowering situation, where power is equitably shared between the professional and the patient. However, the advantage is held by the one with the power-over, and language becomes an important structuring factor in the professional–patient relationship. In public health practice, the advantage is often held by the one with the power-over (the Practitioner) and the language that they choose to use can either strengthen or weaken the professional–client relationship.

The intransitive (indirect) meaning suggests the act of gaining power. This is the litmus test of empowerment because power cannot be given but must be taken by those who seek it. This is a process that can be facilitated by the Practitioner by helping to create the conditions necessary to make it possible for power to be gained. In a professional–patient relationship, this is a mutual role played out by the Practitioner, who facilitates change, and the patient, who identifies and executes the change.

The language used in public health uses both the direct and indirect meanings of power. But in practice, power cannot be given and patients must be enabled by Practitioners to gain power from others. It is the working relationship between Practitioners and patients that is therefore the mechanism to achieve greater control. Box 5.3 shows how the use of language can have both an empowering and a non-empowering effect through the professional–patient relationship. Both accounts (1 and 2) are taken from the same case history file for Beatrice, an imaginary patient.

## Box 5.3 Language and the professional–patient relationship

Which account of Beatrice is more empowering?

Account 1: Beatrice is

- a low-income, single mother;
- unemployed;
- undernourished and anaemic;
- living in a one-room basement apartment;
- looking after two children – her first child was of low birth weight;
- not able to speak English well;
- a smoker and drinks alcohol.

Account 2: Beatrice is

- looking for work that will fit her skills as a trained laboratory technician;
- trying to find ways to supplement her diet but is unable to afford extra money for food shopping;
- living in a small tidy apartment but is looking for better accommodation;
- looking after her two healthy and happy children;
- learning English at night-class but finds it difficult to get a babysitter;
- fluent in Spanish and French;
- trying to give up smoking.

The first account of Beatrice uses a power-over approach in which the Practitioner has presented a series of negative statements about the patient; for example, Beatrice is described as being 'unemployed', 'undernourished' and having 'a low birth weight' child. The first account implies a person who is unhealthy and powerless, and when confronted by such a description, through her contact with different Practitioners and institutions, Beatrice may begin to internalize this description as being true about herself. This is a process that is called learned helplessness (see Chapter 2), a manifestation of power-over the patient by the Practitioner.

In the second account of Beatrice she is portrayed using positive language centred on her own strengths; for example, she is 'trying to give up smoking', 'fluent in French and Spanish' and 'a trained laboratory technician'. This account implies that the patient is struggling but at the same time is trying to help herself and her family. It is a manifestation of power-from-within that offers opportunities to develop an empowering professional–patient relationship. In a public health system that is sensitive to vulnerability in society, the negative description of Beatrice (account 1) may actually be more empowering. The system is designed to respond to Beatrice's vulnerability and may be more likely to provide her with support from social and welfare services, for example, to find employment, childcare and better housing. The positive description of Beatrice (account 2) on the other hand may result in her needs being given a lower priority within a system that has limited resources and assesses her as not being at any immediate risk.

Technical terms are also a part of the everyday language of Practitioners, for example, medical diagnostic vocabulary, and have evolved as knowledge has developed within professional groups. However, the use of specialist language is often confusing to lay people or even to other professionals. The use of terms such as 'high risk' and 'target group' also imply passivity and locate the problem with the client rather than as a relationship to the influence of broader determinants. While it may sometimes be necessary to use specific technical terms, the professional–patient relationship is more empowering when it uses a language that is understood by everyone. To build the power-from-within of their patients the Practitioner must relinquish some control over their use of technical language and engage in a more empowering dialogue. In practice, an empowering professional language means that the Practitioners should be aware of the influence of their professional language and technical terms and be sensitive to the perceptions of patients.

## Salutogenesis and patient empowerment

The term 'salutogenesis' was developed by Aaron Antonovsky during his studies of how people, including patients, manage stress, recover and stay well. Antonovsky observed that while many people suffered from stress, not all people or patients had negative health outcomes and some people actually achieved good health despite their exposure to potentially disabling stress factors. A stress factor was pathogenic, neutral or salutary depending on Generalized Resistance Resources (GRRs). A GRR is any coping resource that is effective in avoiding or combating a range of psychosocial stressors, for example, finances, power-from-within and social support. The GRRs can therefore enable patients to better manage stressful events in their lives in relation to the Sense of Coherence (SOC): an orientation that expresses the extent to which one has pervasive, enduring, though dynamic, feelings of confidence (Antonovsky, 1979, p. 123). The SOC has three components: 1. Comprehensibility: a belief that things happen in an orderly and predictable fashion and a sense that you can understand events in your life and reasonably predict what will happen in the future; 2. Manageability: a belief that you have the skills or ability, the support, the help or the resources necessary to take care of things, and that things are manageable and within your control; 3. Meaningfulness: a belief that things in life are interesting and a source of satisfaction, that things are really worth it and that there is good reason or purpose to care about what happens. The third element, meaningfulness, is felt to be the most important. If a patient believes there is no reason to persist and survive and confront challenges, if they have no sense of meaning, then they will have no motivation to comprehend and manage stressful events (Lindstrom and Eriksson, 2005). Strategies that can strengthen a patient's power-from-within (Chapter 4) or support patient self-help groups (Chapter 6) will help them to be more motivated to manage stressful events in their lives. In comparison with concepts such as resilience (where the conditions and mechanisms are more rigid and contextual), salutogenesis therefore has its strength in adaptability and as an approach towards focusing on problem solving to manage stressful situations.

## Patient action

Patient empowerment involves both individual self-care and the broader collective action to enable patients and their carers to have more of an influence on health service delivery. Patient advocacy, for example, can play an important role in enabling people to have more influence on services that do not meet their needs or expectations and to represent themselves, and others, to speak out about their rights.

## Patient advocacy

Advocacy involves people acting on behalf of themselves or on behalf of others to argue a position and to influence the outcome of decisions (Smithies and Webster, 1998). The different forms of patient action, for example, patient involvement action groups, use advocacy to help patients, family members and health professionals to speak and act on behalf of others, or on their own behalf. Advocacy uses a variety of tactics that include media campaigns, public speaking and commissioning and publishing research with the intention of influencing policy, resource allocation and decision making within political and social systems. Media advocacy, for example, aims to get the media's attention and to frame the needs of patients in an appropriate way so that policy makers, politicians and the public understand the issue. Media advocacy targets the ways in which issues come to be regarded as newsworthy to help set the discussion and to try to influence the boundaries within which the debate can take place. This can have an influence on what the media sets as its agenda which can be potentially very powerful for patient advocacy groups.

Patient advocates may be an individual or an organization, they can address a number of issues and may express patient needs about health care and service delivery. Typical patient advocacy activities include human rights, matters of privacy, confidentiality or informed consent, patient representation, education, survivors and the support of family carers. Patient advocates give a 'voice' to patients but also aim to inform the public, the political and regulatory world, health care providers, professional associations and the private sector, including the pharmaceutical industry. Patient advocacy activities can begin from the concerns raised by patient self-help groups, networks and action groups or from the efforts of individual patients, carers and survivors. The Nottingham Advocacy Group (NAG), for example, was established in the mid-1980s in the UK. The group grew out of meetings held by patients on hospital wards to develop a good relationship with the service provider. While involved in the personal development of its members, the main aim of the group was to advocate for improvements in mental health policy and service delivery. The NAG also supported the development of similar groups, but as patient involvement became more accepted as part of official policy, its contract with the local Trust was offered to other groups and the NAG had to review its role as an advocate for patients in a changing and competitive environment (Barnes and Gell, 2011).

The patient's limitations and the limits of the care that family members can provide, as well as the limits of health care services, can result in specific needs having to be addressed both in society and in institutional contexts, such as hospitals. Networks and action groups can therefore also play a role in advocating for patients, their carers and for health professionals to better meet their needs and to be able to speak out about their rights. I next discuss the importance of patient networks and of patient involvement action groups in empowerment.

## Patient networks

A network is a structure of relationships, both personal and professional, through which individuals maintain and receive emotional support, resources, services and information for the improvement of their health and well-being. Networks set a context within groups, formal organizations and institutions for those who work in or are served by them, which, in turn, affects what people do, how they feel and what happens to them (Wright, 1997).

A network is a structure of relationships linking social actors that in turn are the building blocks of human experience, mapping the connections that individuals have to one another (Pescosolido, 1991). Social structures are not based therefore on categorizations such as age, gender or race but on the actual nature of the social contacts that individuals have and their impact on people's lives (White, 1992).

A patient network can be formed by its members for the benefit of its members, both patients and health practitioners, and can be the means through which people can become empowered through better communication and organizational structures. Patient Concern (UK), for example, operates a network in collaboration with other active groups run by patients and volunteers on issues that matter to them, including protection for whistle-blowers, assisted suicide, campaigns against the reduction of hospital beds and strengthening complaints procedures (Patient Concern, 2012).

Networks can be an indication of related health behaviour; for example, people who experience the weight gain of others in their social networks may then more readily accept weight gain in themselves. Moreover, social distance is more important than geographic distance within networks and is an important role for a process involving the induction and person-to-person spread of obesity. Peer support interventions that allow for a modification of people's social networks are therefore more successful than those that do not and can be used to also spread positive health behaviours because people's perceptions of their own risk of illness may depend on the people around them (Christakis and Fowler, 2007).

Networks have some features that are particularly relevant to professional groups whose functions rely on the interactions between a network's members. Social relationships underpin network activity with a strong sense of professional identity and solidarity and offer individuals and organizations the opportunity to access complementary resources and expertise. The Patients Association (UK), for example, is a network about common patient issues for better information and support. The most frequent complaints received by the Patients Association concern poor communication, toileting, pain relief, nutrition and hydration. The Patients Association addresses the shared concerns of its members including the 'duty to refer', to ensure they are getting access to the best treatment (Patients Association, 2015). Access to information is the best way to make sure this is happening and patient support groups are ideally placed to provide this service. Practitioners cannot be experts in all fields and so it is important for them to be able to direct patients to other organizations which have the expertise. Practitioners can then actively support patients in finding support groups that could help them with managing their condition.

## Patient involvement action groups

Patient involvement action groups (PIAGs) involve patients acting on behalf of themselves or on behalf of others to argue a position and to influence the outcome of decisions. PIAGs use tactics that include media campaigns, demonstrations and petitions with the intention of influencing policy, resource allocation and decision making within health systems. PIAGs promote health care rights as well as trying to enhance health initiatives for the availability, safety and quality of care.

There is an important distinction to be made between PIAGs that are supported by a health service provider, and those that are independent and are formed by patients, for the benefit of their members. In practice both health service providers and patients can work together because the PIAGs can help to establish priorities and to provide a platform for testing and modifying plans. Patients are encouraged and supported by PIAGs to take more responsibility for their own health by increasing health literacy, raising awareness of lifestyle options and promoting self-care, particularly for minor everyday illnesses. PIAGs may also promote broader support, such as arranging transport for disabled patients, or by running self-help activities, such as weight management sessions. When establishing a PIAG it is important to develop a plan for setting up and developing the group with clear goals that must be taken seriously by the health care service to help to promote its activities, the issues it raises and the plans that have been developed. Inevitably, there can be problems when establishing PIAGs; for example, members of the group may have unrealistic expectations, it may be unrepresentative or it may develop into a complaints forum rather than a means for sharing constructive ideas. However, the advantages of the PIAG are that patient satisfaction is improved, costs reduced, services improved and resources used more efficiently, as well as patients having a real sense of ownership in the changes that are made in the health care system (Tidy, 2015).

One PIAG in a UK hospital was established to allow concerns to be raised anonymously and to obtain feedback about actions taken. Patients and their carers were given comment forms which could be returned to a member of staff or placed in a collection box. Once a month all of the comments, both positive and negative, were reviewed by the group, and action was decided upon at an appropriate level, or a report given about action already taken. The results of each action were posted on display boards in the wards to inform the patients and their carers of the actions taken. These actions included side rooms for infection control to be fitted with curtains to act as a screen, wards which suffered from solar glare to receive vertical blinds and shelves to be put up in bathrooms to help patients to manage their own personal belongings. Each ward was asked to nominate representatives, of whom one would be available to attend each monthly meeting. The number of formal complaints decreased to less than 20% of the previous level, as patients gained confidence that their comments would be acted upon and that the hospital environment had improved (Improvement Network, 2011).

The predominant view of patient empowerment is an individualistic approach that gives credibility to what the individual has to offer self-care. However, patient empowerment should involve both strengthening individual power-from-within and broader collective action. The goals of patient empowerment are to give patients more control over self-care as well as to enable them collectively to have more of an influence on the health care that they receive and towards which they are increasingly expected to contribute. Most importantly, patients must be given the ability to take action on their own behalf, and on the behalf of others, if the health care system does not meet their needs and expectations.

Next, in Chapter 6 I discuss working with groups as an important means of helping others to become more critically aware of their circumstances. Group work offers the opportunity for people to find a 'voice', to develop their skills and to work with others to achieve their goals.

# HELPING GROUPS TO BE MORE CRITICAL

Working with groups is an important part of public health practice because this is often the point at which individuals are able to progress to collective action. Small groups allow people to become better organized and mobilized towards addressing their needs. Working with groups also provides an opportunity for the Practitioner to assist others to develop stronger social links and skills, and to raise the resources necessary to support their actions. Group members usually begin with a focus on their immediate needs, but with an increase in knowledge and capacity this can shift towards broader empowerment issues, such as health inequality and social injustice.

## The link between education and empowerment

The link between education and empowerment involves more than simply acquiring new knowledge. Knowledge can actually lead to a greater sense of disempowerment when a person is unable to use this information to improve their circumstances. The link between education and empowerment relates to critical education, a concept that was used by Paulo Freire, through his ideas on empowerment, to build awareness in literacy programmes for the impoverished in Brazil in the 1950s. The central premise is that education is not neutral but is influenced by the context of one's life. To Freire, the purpose of education is liberation, in which people become the subjects of their own learning, involving a critical reflection and analysis of their personal circumstances. To achieve this, Freire proposed a group dialogue approach to share ideas and experiences and to promote critical thinking by posing problems to allow people to uncover the root causes of their powerlessness and poverty. This is an ongoing interaction between the Practitioner and their client in a cycle of action/reflection/action. Once critically aware, people can then plan more effective actions to change their circumstances. It should be noted that this approach involves a commitment by the individual to understand the causes of inequality and to develop realistic actions to resolve the situation.

A key consideration when educating adolescents is the age at which they begin to understand their world in a concrete and abstract way, such that they can fully engage with critical education. An approach based on their right to participate as social actors accepts that they act on the world around them. Practitioners can then engage with adolescents about their worlds and involve them in identifying their needs and in decision making processes. Although there is not a definitive youngest age at which adolescents can be engaged to empower themselves, a guide of 14 years, give or take a year, depending on the individual and the socio-cultural context, can be used in public health practice (Laverack, 2013).

## Increasing critical awareness

Critical awareness can be described as the ability to reflect on the assumptions underlying our actions and to contemplate better ways of living (Goodman et al., 1998). Groups cannot intentionally empower themselves without having an understanding of the underlying causes of their powerlessness. This may occur from within the group, often developing slowly, and may be facilitated through a process that promotes discussion, reflection and action. This is called 'critical consciousness' or 'conscientization' and involves learning using 'empowerment education' as developed by Paulo Freire (Freire, 2005). Increasing critical awareness involves people developing realistic actions to begin to resolve the conditions that have created their powerlessness in the first place (Nutbeam, 2000). Increasing critical awareness can be enhanced by Practitioners by using approaches that achieve stronger social support and skills development, including lay epidemiology, self-help groups, photo-voice, health literacy and strategies for collective decision making. These approaches are discussed next in relation to how Practitioners can help to increase the critical awareness of others in their everyday work.

## Lay epidemiology

Lay epidemiology describes the processes by which people in their everyday lives can more critically understand and interpret health risks (Allmark and Tod, 2006). To reach conclusions about the risks to their health, people access information from a variety of sources, including the mass media, the internet, friends and family. Lay epidemiology presents a challenge to the accepted wisdom of the health professions as people use this information to critically assess their situation in at least two ways:

1  People, in reaching their conclusions, do not necessarily accept health messages. People have recognized that some health messages are 'half-truths' and this is further confused by the changing of some messaging, for example, in regard to safe limits for alcohol consumption. The prevention paradox refers to targeting the behaviour of the majority who are at a low to medium risk, which has little effect at the individual level. For example, reducing dietary fat consumption for the whole population would reduce coronary heart disease but it is difficult to change the behaviour of those whose risk is only low to medium. Practitioners have therefore chosen to use simple messaging that does not tell the whole truth by exaggerating the risks of a particular behaviour or the benefits of changing that behaviour. A reliance on information-based approaches has led to mistrust, and when people feel that the risk does not apply to them, they may choose to reject the advice given (Hunt and Emslie, 2001).
2  People have cultural and personal values that undermine the meaning of health messages; for example, a person can choose not to give up smoking on the basis that, although it may be damaging to their health, they believe that the benefits of smoking, such as reducing stress, outweigh the risk. People's perception of risk depends on their circumstances, culture and values and this can be in contrast to traditional public health approaches, which are usually empirically derived (Allmark and Tod, 2006).

Attempts by authorities to manipulate the public can lead to dissatisfied people using lay epidemiology as a pathway for community-based empowerment. For example, in the UK public concerns were raised about the measles, mumps and rubella vaccine. The public health authorities saw this as an effective option with few side effects. However, following media reports of conflicting scientific evidence, the public became increasingly concerned that the vaccine could lead to bowel disease and autism. These concerns were further confounded by the public's past distrust over the mishandling of the outbreak of 'mad cow disease' (bovine spongiform encephalopathy or BSE) and conflicting evidence on the benefits of screening, for example, the benefits of mammography (Smith, 2002).

The means of governing people is dependent on expert systems of knowledge, science and empirical truths. This is the means to regulate how professionals are given more control over health care, knowledge and even issues that do not necessarily fall within the bio-medical sphere. The public health view has historically held unquestioned wisdom, but in a postmodern world there is no one truth, whether defined by public health or any other experts. There are different opinions based on different views and theories, none of which hold an absolute truth. Lay epidemiology can pose a threat to public health because it challenges the accepted wisdom, which is then no longer the dominant perspective (Brown and Zavestoski, 2004). However, the public is open to rational discussion and Practitioners are right to engage with them to offer advice that is based on sound scientific evidence. Public health practitioners have therefore played an important mediating role between those in authority, the public and social organizations, documenting and establishing trends based on rationality. This sets standards of normality that can build upon political policies and create opportunities to show how public health can overcome particular issues using its expert and legitimate power. Public health can therefore be a coercive force to influence the way people think and act (Lupton, 1995) that is not always intentional on the part of the Practitioners, who face the challenge of meeting targets based on bio-medical outcomes and which the public may not be willing to engage with. The danger is that public health can present an illusion of greater individual and collective choice while acting to hide an agenda that intends to control others to do what we as professionals want them to do, even against their will. Public health then becomes the very opposite of an empowering practice.

## Self-help groups

Self-help groups organize around a specific and shared need in which the members are usually supportive of one another and are often managed by the participants (Laverack, 2009). Self-help is a self-guided improvement, normally for economic, intellectual or emotional purposes. Self-help utilizes support groups using either face-to-face or online services to provide friendship, emotional support, experiential knowledge and a greater sense of belonging. Self-help groups can be used to learn about health, to acquire skills and to provide peer support, for example, weight loss groups or Alcoholics Anonymous. The group locale provides an opportunity for the Practitioner to assist others to develop stronger social support and to mobilize resources. Self-help groups, therefore, are useful to bring people together and help them to identify needs which they feel are important. Needs assessment skills are necessary to be able to do this, and when these are not present within the group the role of the Practitioner is to assist the group to build its capacity.

The importance of participating in groups can be illustrated by the setting up of women's groups in a rural population in Nepal, which led to a reduction in neonatal and maternal mortality. By participating in groups the women were better able to define, analyse and then, through the support of others, articulate and act on their concerns around childbirth. The advantage of the participation was that it strengthened social networks and improved social support between the women and between the women and the providers of the health care services (Manandhar et al., 2004). There is also strong evidence that community mobilization is an effective method for promoting participation and empowering communities with a wide range of benefits, such as cost-effectiveness, reductions in mortality and improvements in the health of newborn infants, children and mothers. Nonetheless, community mobilization and participation are often not a feature of most large-scale, top-down public health programmes (Rosato et al., 2008).

Self-help groups often have limited resources and because of their small size their inclusion in the policy process can lead to them being absorbed by it unless they are able to grow and develop into broader community-based organizations (Allsop et al., 2004). The challenge is to enable people to move forward from individual issues, to be included in small groups and then to develop into broader community-based organizations. This progression gives people a greater capacity to work with others who share the same needs and with whom they can collectively take the necessary actions to resolve their needs. Box 6.1 provides specific criteria for selecting and working with groups based on the principles of an empowering public health practice.

---

### Box 6.1 Criteria for selecting groups

1  The group has unmet needs

   ▶ groups that are dysfunctional or unorganized
   ▶ groups that are neglected by other service providers, politicians, the media
   ▶ groups experiencing serious disadvantages
   ▶ groups that don't know how to use the health and welfare system.

2  Our support will have an impact

   ▶ the group is able to identify its goals and objectives and to focus on a need
   ▶ the group is able to organize itself and its own activities
   ▶ leadership arises within the group
   ▶ there is a sufficient membership within the group that some success will be likely
   ▶ the group is able to achieve some short-term, visible successes
   ▶ there is a sizeable number of people whose health will be affected positively by the group's success.

3  A new group needs to be organized

   ▶ there are no other agencies better able to do the organizing
   ▶ there is a critical mass of individuals who express interest in meeting as a group
   ▶ there is health institution support and clear decision making to do the organizing

*(Continued)*

> ▶ there is positive group dynamics
> ▶ the group develops a sense of responsibility for its own actions.

4   I have knowledge or skills relevant to the group's needs

5   The group will grow and become autonomous

> ▶ the group knows or learns its rights, privileges and responsibilities
> ▶ the group is or can become independent of the health agencies
> ▶ the group is able to negotiate its own terms with health agencies
> ▶ the group learns how to look for, and use, resources from within and from government.

6   The group is open in membership and accountable to those it claims to represent

> ▶ the group is inclusive (open to anyone who wants to join)
> ▶ the group is able to develop some means to be accountable to those whom it claims to represent
> ▶ the accountability involves all members.

7   The group is internally democratic

> ▶ the group does not use unilateral decision making
> ▶ the group does not censor opposition within the group
> ▶ the group does not control information
> ▶ the group does not exclude others from leadership positions
> ▶ the group does not have hierarchical forms of organization.

Source: adapted from Labonté (1998).

# Photo-voice

Photo-voice is a process by which people can identify, represent and enhance their critical awareness through a specific photographic technique. Photo-voice provides people with cameras to enable them to act as recorders and potential catalysts for social action and change in their own communities. It uses the immediacy of the visual image and accompanying stories to provide anecdotal evidence of what really matters to people at the community level. Photo-voice has two main goals:

1   to enable people to record and reflect their community's strengths and concerns;
2   to promote critical awareness and dialogue about personal and community issues through group discussions using photographs.

Photo-voice engages people in a three-stage process that provides the foundation for analysing the visual images that they have created:

Stage 1. Selecting: The group chooses those photographs that most accurately reflect the community's concerns, based on what is most significant in the images.
Stage 2. Contextualizing or story telling: This occurs in the group discussions, suggested by the acronym VOICE: voicing our individual and collective experience. Photographs alone, considered outside the context of their own stories, can contradict

the essence of photo-voice. People therefore describe and share the meaning of the images in group discussions.

**Stage 3. Codifying:** The participatory approach can give multiple meanings to singular images and thus frames the third stage, codifying. In this stage, participants may identify three types of dimensions that arise from the dialogue process: issues, themes or theories. The group codifies issues when the concerns targeted for action are pragmatic, immediate and tangible and are the most direct application of the analysis. The group can also codify themes and patterns, or develop theories that are grounded in a more systematic analysis of the images.

Photo-voice is used to reach, inform and organize community members, enabling them to prioritize their concerns and discuss problems and solutions. Photo-voice goes beyond the conventional role of needs assessment by inviting people to promote their own and their community's well-being. It is a method that enables people to define for themselves and for others, including policy makers, what is worth remembering and what needs to be changed (PhotoVoice, 2015). Box 6.2 provides a case study that illustrates how photo-voice can be used in a practical setting to address the issue of maternal and child health.

---

**Box 6.2 Photo-voice for maternal and child health**

Contra Costa is a large, economically and ethnically diverse county in the San Francisco Bay area in the USA. Sixty county residents aged 13–50 participated in three sessions during which they received training from the local health department in the techniques and process of photo-voice. Residents were provided with disposable cameras and were encouraged to take photographs reflecting their views on family, maternal and child health assets and concerns in their community, and then participated in group discussions about their photographs. Community events were held to enable participants to educate maternal and child health (MCH) staff and community leaders.

Results: The photo-voice project provided MCH staff with information to supplement existing quantitative perinatal data and contributed to an understanding of key MCH issues that participating community residents wanted to see addressed. Participants' concerns centred on the need for safe places for children's recreation and for improvement in the broader community environment within county neighbourhoods. Participants' definitions of family, maternal and child health assets and concerns differed from those that MCH professionals may typically view as MCH issues (low birth weight, maternal mortality, teen pregnancy prevention), which helped MCH program staff to expand priorities and include residents' foremost concerns.

Conclusions: MCH professionals can apply photo-voice as an innovative participatory research methodology to engage community members in needs assessment, asset mapping and program planning, and in reaching policy makers to advocate strategies promoting family, maternal and child health as informed from a grassroots perspective (Wang and Pies, 2004).

# Health literacy

Health literacy is a repackaging of the relationship between education and empowerment. It grew out of the realization that interventions that had relied too heavily on communication had failed to achieve substantial results (Nutbeam, 2000). What is new about health literacy, therefore, is that health education becomes more than just the transmission of information and uses skills development and confidence building to help people to make better-informed decisions that will allow them to gain greater control over their lives (Renkert and Nutbeam, 2001). Health literacy enables people to gain access to, understand and use information in ways that promote and maintain good health (World Health Organization, 1998). Health literacy is first dependent on the level of basic literacy in the community, that is, the ability to read and write in everyday life. In practice it can be delivered at three levels:

1 **Basic/functional literacy** – sufficient basic skills in reading and writing to be able to function effectively in everyday situations, broadly compatible with the narrow definition.
2 **Communicative/interactive literacy** – more advanced cognitive and literacy skills, which, together with social skills, can be used to actively participate in everyday activities, to extract information and derive meaning from different forms of communication, and to apply new information to changing circumstances.
3 **Critical literacy** – more advanced cognitive skills, which, together with social skills, can be applied to critically analyse information, and to use this information to exert greater control over life events and situations (Nutbeam, 2000).

The challenge in public health practice is to achieve critical health literacy because the value of health literacy is as a tool to help Practitioners to become more effective communicators by increasing the critical awareness of their clients. In a public health practice dominated by communication, health literacy offers an advanced approach that enables people to better understand how to take individual and collective action. In Box 6.3 I provide the example of using health literacy to improve antenatal care.

---

### Box 6.3 Health literacy and antenatal classes

A potential use of health literacy is for the development of antenatal classes to provide women with the cognitive and social skills to maintain their health and that of their children. Women attending antenatal classes are often highly motivated and literate. But antenatal classes are sometimes constrained by time, and the natural curiosity and anxiety of the women make it difficult to transfer all the necessary information and skills. Classes therefore focus on the transfer of factual information rather than on decision making skills for childbirth and parenting, which can require more time. The latter is empowering rather than just passive and central to health literacy techniques that focus on providing the necessary skills and enabling women to make informed choices. Using this empowering approach means that the entire content of the antenatal class would not have to be delivered, reducing the time needed for teaching and providing more time to allow the mothers to ask questions and to discuss issues (Renkert and Nutbeam, 2001).

## Strategies for collective decision making

Strategies for better decision making about different health options can be an empowering tool for Practitioners to use when working with groups. Decision making is a highly complex procedure and a practical approach to promote the principles of this process is outlined below. I use the example of helping a group to develop decision making skills that will give its members more control over their desire to improve their health over a six month period.

### Step 1: Ranking key options

The group first makes a list of the key options covering their particular health concern. The Practitioner can help by providing specific technical information in response to questions about the issue and by helping the participants to rank their options. The ranking must come from the group without being coerced by the Practitioner. If the number of ranked options is large, the Practitioner can assist the group to produce a prioritized list; for example, a ranked list to improve health in the next six months might include:

> 1  To stop smoking.
> 2  To do more exercise.
> 3  To lose weight.
> 4  To eat more healthily.

A ranking of the different choices as set out in step 1 is in itself insufficient to help others to empower themselves. This information must also be transformed into decisions and actions which is achieved through developing a decision making matrix for positive changes in the prioritized areas using:

> Step 2. Decisions on the key actions to be taken;
> Step 3. Decisions on the key activities for each action taken; and
> Step 4. The identification of resources.

### Step 2: Decisions on the key actions to be taken

The group is next asked to decide on how the situation can be improved for each ranked issue. The purpose is to first identify the most feasible actions that will improve the present situation and then to provide a more detailed strategy in step 3 outlining the activities. This information is placed in column 2 of the decision making matrix shown in Table 6.1.

Taking the first ranked health option in step 1 (To stop smoking), the decisions on the key actions to be taken might include:

> ▶ Remove all cigarettes from the home and workplace.
> ▶ Attend motivation classes to help to stop smoking.
> ▶ Use a substitute for smoking, such as e-cigarettes or nicotine patches.

## Step 3: Decisions on the key activities for each action taken

The group is next asked to consider the most feasible actions that can be carried out in practice and, in particular, to sequence activities in order to make an improvement and to set a realistic time frame. These are placed in column 3 of the matrix. Continuing from the example in step 2, the activities to implement the identified actions to stop smoking might include the following:

> ▶ Collect all cigarettes in house and dispose of them.
> ▶ Do not purchase any more cigarettes.
> ▶ Identify local classes or start a new class. Make time to attend one class per week. Identify a friend to attend initial classes for support.
> ▶ Discuss best alternative products with a doctor or pharmacist. Make an appointment to speak with a doctor in the next seven days.
> ▶ Buy alternative products and use for the next three to six months.

## Step 4: Identification of resources

The group next identifies the resources that are necessary to implement the actions in steps 2 and 3. The Practitioner can help the group to map the necessary resources, for example, information, finances and social support. To undertake the actions to stop smoking might include the following resources:

> ▶ The availability of local self-motivation class.
> ▶ Money to pay for classes and time to attend the classes.
> ▶ Access to a pharmacy or Practitioner to discuss the best options for a smoking substitute.
> ▶ Money to purchase smoking cessation aids and alternative products.

## The decision making matrix

The strategy for decision making can be represented by using a simplified matrix as shown in Table 6.1, in which the ranked health issue is placed in the left-hand column followed by sequential columns for the key decisions, key activities and resources. The matrix provides a summary of the decisions, actions and resources to be undertaken and is the basis for an 'informal contract' between the Practitioner and the group members. It identifies specific tasks or responsibilities, usually set against a time frame; for example, the time frame to stop smoking was given as six months. It also identifies the resources that will be required to fulfil these tasks and responsibilities, within the agreed time frame, by both the Practitioner and the group members.

It is crucial that Practitioners are sensitive to their position and status and the influence that these can have on their clients. It is important that they understand the influence of their professional language and the technical terms that they use (see Chapter 5) and continuously appraise their own professional behaviour. Such awareness is termed a reflexive practice that allows Practitioners to be more critical about the way they use

**Table 6.1**   The decision making matrix: Stop smoking in the next six months

| Step 1. Priority | Step 2. Key decisions | Step 3. Key activities | Step 4. Resources |
|---|---|---|---|
| To stop smoking in the next six months. | Remove all cigarettes from the home and workplace.<br><br>Attend motivation classes to help to stop smoking.<br><br>Use a substitute for smoking, such as chewing gum or nicotine patches. | Collect all cigarettes in house and dispose of them.<br>Do not purchase any more cigarettes.<br><br>Identify local classes. Make time to attend one class per week. Identify a friend to attend initial classes for support.<br><br>Discuss best alternative products with a doctor or pharmacist. Make an appointment to speak with a doctor in the next seven days.<br><br>Buy alternative products from the pharmacy and use as prescribed for the next three to six months. | The availability of local self-motivation class.<br><br>Money to pay for classes and time to attend the classes.<br><br>Access to a pharmacy or Practitioner to discuss the best options for a smoking substitute.<br><br>Money to purchase smoking cessation aids or substitute products. |

their knowledge and power to have a professional influence over others, including other professionals and their clients (Laverack, 2009).

Next, in Chapter 7 I discuss those aspects of empowerment that enhance the ability of communities to better organize and mobilize themselves towards gaining power. I first clarify the concept of 'community' and community engagement and then offer a five-point framework for helping communities to become empowered, including a discussion on the role of health social movements in public health practice.

# 7

# HELPING COMMUNITIES TO BECOME EMPOWERED

Helping communities to become empowered involves two fundamental issues: capacity building and collective action. To better understand how a more empowering approach to public health practice can be applied in this context it is important to first consider the characteristics of a community.

## What is a 'community'?

It is important for Practitioners to think beyond the customary view of a community as a place where people live, such as a village or a neighbourhood. These locales can be an aggregate of non-connected people, especially in an urban context, within which interest groups form. Geographic communities therefore often consist of heterogeneous individuals and groups with changing and dynamic social relations. The diversity of people's interests within a geographic community can create problems with regard to the selection of representation of its members (Zakus and Lysack, 1998). Practitioners need to carefully consider who the legitimate representatives of a community are. Those individuals who have the energy, time and motivation to become involved in activities may, in fact, not be supported by everyone and may be considered as acting out of self-interest. In these circumstances, a dominant minority may dictate what the community needs are, unless adequate actions are taken to involve everyone. The key characteristics of a community are provided in Box 7.1 and include aspects of spatial location, social dimension and need.

---

**Box 7.1 The key characteristics of a 'community'**

1 A spatial dimension, that is, a place or locale.
2 Non-spatial dimensions (interests, issues, identities) that involve people who otherwise make up heterogeneous and disparate groups.
3 Social interactions that are dynamic and bind people into relationships with one another.
4 Identification of shared needs and concerns that can be achieved through a process of collective action. (Laverack, 2004, p. 46)

---

Within geographic or spatial dimensions multiple communities can exist and individuals may belong to several different interest groups at the same time. Interest groups exist as a legitimate means by which individuals can find a means of expression and are able to participate in a more formal way through committees, social clubs and associations. Interest groups provide the opportunity for people to collectively address mutual concerns, such as the members of a smoking cessation club or a local action group. A group setting provides individuals with a means through which they can take a step closer towards achieving collective action by participating with others who share the same concerns as themselves. The challenge to public health is how to engage with individuals, interest groups and communities within a programme context.

Community engagement is a collaborative process, often between an outside agency and the community, involving identifying problem-solving solutions to issues that affect people's lives. Community engagement begins with people becoming better informed about issues that affect them and how they can become involved in addressing them. The best approach is to use a 'facilitated dialogue' between the community and the outside agents to allow the knowledge and priorities of both to decide an appropriate direction for the programme. A needs assessment undertaken by community members can also strengthen their role in the design of the programme (Laverack, 2007). Next, I provide the findings of a study to identify common themes for community engagement, in this case with Chinese migrants, in regard to accidents and injuries in the home setting.

## Engaging Chinese communities

Adopting a new lifestyle can result in accidents and injuries, yet Asian migrants in New Zealand were found to have little understanding of their entitlements to accident insurance cover, the health care system and rehabilitation services. For example, in 2006 only 4.6% of Asians in New Zealand claimed for accident entitlements, well below the national average (Accident Compensation Corporation, 2006). A qualitative study into engaging with Chinese communities to help prevent injuries found four common themes among recent Chinese migrants in Auckland (Tse et al., 2011):

**Theme 1: Resettlement and relocation issues**
Recently arrived Chinese migrants had different experiences and lifestyles in their country of origin. A lack of familiarity with the New Zealand lifestyle and limited knowledge of how to cater for different circumstances created a tendency for accidents and injuries to occur on a more regular basis.

**Theme 2: Lack of communication**
Some Chinese migrants were confused about the function and services provided by the government and attributed this to a lack of communication or the lack of such a service in their home country. Prior to sustaining an injury, most migrants knew about a rehabilitation service by name; however, at the time of injury they were not confident about accessing services. Language barriers and a lack of resources translated into Chinese were identified as reasons in failing to engage with local services.

**Theme 3: Deployment of Chinese media**
Chinese migrants suggested a variety of channels through which their community could be better informed about available services, with an emphasis on utilizing Chinese media, Chinese newspapers, radio stations and websites, and holding workshops.

**Theme 4: Community readiness and building community capacity**
Joining one or more community organizations is an ordinary practice for Chinese migrants, particularly new migrants, who have a great deal of trust and confidence in these organizations. Reasons identified in the study for using Chinese community-based organizations included socializing, networking, information gathering and preserving

many unique aspects of their culture. To engage with migrants it is therefore important that Practitioners build the capacity of any available community-based organizations.

The four key themes identified in the study highlight some of the difficulties of engaging with migrant communities. In order to effectively engage communities, their voices have to be heard, their needs have to be identified and their capacity has to be developed towards becoming empowered.

## Community empowerment as a five-point continuum

Community empowerment has been consistently viewed in the literature as a five-point continuum comprised of the following elements: personal action; small groups; community organizations; partnerships; and social and political action. This is the continuum model of community empowerment (see Figure 7.1) that represents the potential of people to progress from individual to collective action.

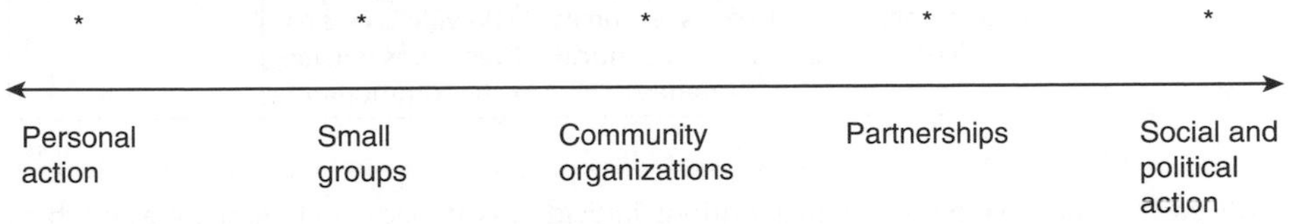

| Personal action | Small groups | Community organizations | Partnerships | Social and political action |

**Figure 7.1**    The continuum of community empowerment (Laverack 1999, p. 92)

The continuum provides a simple, linear interpretation of community empowerment that explains how this concept can be maximized at the personal, organizational and collective levels. Each point on the continuum can be viewed as a progression towards a common goal of community empowerment: social and political change. If a way forward is not possible, stasis occurs or a move back to the preceding point on the continuum. The development of a community organization on the continuum is a pivotal point at which small groups are able to make the transition to a broader structure. It is then through partnerships that organizations are able to gain a greater participant and resource base for their particular cause. The key challenge to Practitioners is how they structure their work with the purpose of assisting others in their progression along the continuum. In Table 7.1 I provide some of the key roles for Practitioners in enabling others to progress along the empowerment continuum. The groups and organizations that arise do have their own dynamics. They may flourish for a time, then fade away for reasons as much to do with changes in the people, as with a lack of broader political or financial support. Public health practice is a part of this dynamic, an important part that, as I explain in this book, can help others to become more empowered.

### Individual empowerment for personal action

A personal action to improve health can begin when individuals feel powerless about a situation, feel the desire to rectify what they perceive as an unjust situation, or want to take action in response to an emotive experience in their lives. For example, a person may become active in a community support group for neighbourhood safety following an assault on them in a public place. This helps the person to come to terms with the event and also allows them to start to work towards having a broader influence, for example, on improved policing, street lighting and public transport in their neighbourhood. In a programme context, the basis for personal action is often developed during the planning phase, for example, through a needs assessment and later developed as a part of the broader objectives.

Table 7.1    Key enabling roles for Practitioners

| Personal action | Small groups | Community organizations | Partnerships | Social and political action |
| --- | --- | --- | --- | --- |
| Build a greater sense of control in people's lives by bringing them together in small groups around issues of mutual concern. | Assist the community to identify and prioritize its needs, solutions to the needs and actions to resolve the needs. Strengthen local leadership skills. | Strengthen organizational structures. Link organizations to resources and develop skills to identify, mobilize and access resources. Promote critical awareness. | Develop a shared agenda with other organizations and build local partnerships and alliances between groups. Provide access to resources outside the community. | Provide legitimacy to the concerns raised by others by using their power base and political influence. |

By participating in groups and organizations, individuals can better define, analyse and then, through the support of others, act on their shared concerns. Zakus and Lysack (1998, p. 2) provide a useful definition of participation set in this context as 'the process by which members of the community, either individually or collectively and with varying degrees of commitment, develop their capability to assume greater responsibility for assessing needs, plan and then act to implement their solutions and maintain organizations in support of these efforts'. However, research in the UK has shown that people's willingness to participate in a programme may not be as high as is first reported. For example, of 55% of local residents who said they wanted to participate in a programme directly affecting their community, only 2% actually did participate (Confederation of British Industry, 2006). Engaging with community members to ensure that they fully participate can be a crucial factor in the success or failure of a programme.

Participation is a combination of involvement in decision making mechanisms, accessibility to community organizations and the development of appropriate individual skills, for example, in strategic planning and resource mobilization. Participation strengthens social networks and programmes do have a better chance of success if they involve people in activities rather than delivering them in a top-down approach. Box 7.2 provides some of the main characteristics of participation in helping to empower others for personal action.

## Box 7.2 The characteristics of participation in empowering others

1  A strong participant base involving all stakeholders, including marginalized groups, but sensitive to the cultural and social context.
2  Participants define their own needs, solutions and actions.
3  Participants are involved in decision making mechanisms at planning, implementation and evaluation stages.

*(Continued)*

4 Participants are encouraged to extend into broader issues of the structural causes of powerlessness and to become critically self-aware.

5 Mechanisms exist to allow free flow of information between the different participants through effective communication.

6 Representatives are appointed by members of all groups.

7 The Practitioner fosters an empowering professional–client relationship.

(Laverack, 2007).

## Small groups and empowerment

The involvement in and the development of small groups is often the start of collective action. This locale provides an opportunity for the Practitioner to assist the individual to gain skills, to develop stronger social support and to mobilize resources. Small groups include self-help and interest groups that are organized around a specific issue; for example, 'Quit' is a self-help group for smoking cessation. Community health groups campaign on a specific localized issue, for example, better facilities for the disabled at a health centre. Neighbourhood-based health groups can be started by government agencies to address issues of local concern, such as poor housing, often with an appointed community worker (Jones and Sidell, 1997).

The role of the Practitioner at this point of the continuum is to bring people together and to help them, through a range of participatory techniques, to identify issues which they feel are important. Needs assessment skills are necessary for small groups to be able to identify the common needs of their members, as well as the solutions and actions to resolve their needs. When these skills do not exist or are weak, the role of the Practitioner will be to provide the necessary skills to the community to help it to make an assessment of its own needs (see Chapter 3).

Successful groups often share a number of key characteristics, including elected representatives, meeting on a regular basis, an agreed membership structure (chairperson, secretary, core members), a history of successes that help to build the confidence of the group, keeping records of previous meetings, having financial accounts, the ability to identify and resolve conflicts quickly and to identify the resources available to the group. Small groups often have limited resources and membership and their low level of participation and poor resource base mean that they have little influence (Allsop et al., 2004), and to be successful they must develop into broader community organizations.

## Community organizations and empowerment

Community organizations include committees, co-operatives and associations. They are the organizational elements in which people come together in order to socialize but also to take action to address local and broader concerns. Community organizations are not only larger than small groups but they also have an established structure, more functional leadership, the ability to better organize their members to mobilize resources and to gain the skills that are necessary to make the transition to form partnerships. These skills include planning and strategy development, time management, team building, networking, negotiation, fund-raising, marketing and publicity, and proposal writing. While small groups generally focus inwards on the needs of their members, community organizations focus outwards to the environment that creates those needs in the first place.

A key function of community organizations is to enable people to gain greater access to resources. Internal resources are those raised within the community and include land, food, money, people, skills and local knowledge. External resources are those brought into the community by, for example, the Practitioner, and include financial assistance, technical expertise, knowledge and equipment. The ability of the community to mobilize resources from within and to negotiate resources from beyond itself is an indication of a high degree of organization.

A key role of the Practitioner at this stage of the continuum is to find creative ways to allow others to communicate their ideas and to express their needs. An example of this is the 'toilet festivals' in Mumbai, India (described in Box 7.3), in which settlement dwellers organized themselves and used their resources to draw municipal officials into negotiations.

---

**Box 7.3 The 'toilet festivals' of Mumbai, India**

Community-based organizations set up in the slums of Mumbai, India, identified the problem of poor sanitation and water supply as a key concern to the residents. The organizations developed a strategy to host 'toilet festivals' as official opening ceremonies for sanitary facilities in the community. The press were invited and the usual protocol for a ceremony was observed, with guests invited to attend and banners advertising the event posted. The real purpose of the 'toilet festivals' was to engage with municipal officials, first by demonstrating the initiative of slum dwellers to organize their own construction of sanitary facilities, but second to draw the officials into the debate about the lack of resources and infrastructure. The agenda was re-orientated to include poor living conditions and not solely the previous focus on illegal settlement. The media was able to raise the issue and the slum dwellers were able to short-cut the normal channels of bureaucracy and power-over structures in local government (Appadurai, 2004).

---

The development of community organizations and local leadership are closely connected. Leadership requires a strong participant base just as community organizations require the direction and structure of strong leadership (Goodman et al., 1998). Anderson et al. (2006) found that people with a shared commitment to public involvement were important to motivate others in the community and to develop partnerships. Local people were drawn into the process of participation and with increased confidence and capacity became powerful advocates for their community. A proper balance between professional inputs and lay people was seen as essential because conflict was found to occur when there was a lack of clarity regarding who was in control of the programme. When leaders are not able to provide a direction, the role of the Practitioner is to help develop their skills, for example, in management and strategic planning.

The Practitioner should carefully consider who represents the 'community', how they are selected, their existing level of training and what the balance is between their economic and traditional influence in the community. The problem of selecting appropriate leadership is discussed by Goodman et al. (1998), who argue that a pluralistic approach in the community, one where there is an interplay between the positional leaders, those who have been elected or appointed, and the reputed leaders, those who informally serve the community, has a better chance of success. The dominance of one leader can result in them using this power to manipulate situations for their own self-interest. To illustrate this I provide an example in Box 7.4 of how local leaders can misrepresent the interests of their community.

### Box 7.4 Misrepresentation by local leadership

Lucy Earle et al. (2004, p. 27), a community development researcher and her colleagues, provide an example of the manipulation of programmes by local leaders in Central Asia. The village leader in one community had used his influence to obtain assistance from an NGO to help provide irrigation pipes and an electric pump to improve the water supply of the community. But not all members of the community were satisfied with these developments, especially groups of low-income women. The water supplied was too expensive for them and the pipes were laid to better serve the family members of the village leader. However, they could not complain because to contradict the leader could mean serious consequences for the livelihoods of poor families; for example, the village leader provided temporary employment during harvest and distributed flour to poorer residents. Not only did the leader hold an influential position in the community but his sons also held posts in the local government administration. The village leader was able to use his power-over others in the community, mostly over marginalized groups, to manipulate the distribution of resources and gain access to decision making processes.

## Partnerships and empowerment

To be effective in influencing decision making, community organizations must link with others sharing similar concerns. The purpose of developing partnerships is to allow local organizations to grow beyond their own concerns and to take a stronger position through networking and resource mobilization. The key challenge is to remain focused on the concern that brings the groups together and not on the individual needs of the different groups in the partnership. Box 7.5 provides an example of the Altogether Better project, a collaborative partnership for community capacity building in the UK.

### Box 7.5 The Altogether Better project

The Altogether Better project is a collaborative partnership aimed at building capacity to empower communities to improve their own health and well-being. The overall aim of the 'I Am My Community' project was to build capacity in communities and to extend the skills and expertise of local volunteers. The project was undertaken in two disadvantaged communities in Sheffield, UK: Firth Park and

*(Continued)*

Sharrow. Four main practical lessons emerged: 1. the importance of securing adequate financial resources to pay for the staff involved, which proved to be very time intensive; 2. the need to involve a wider pool of volunteers to expand the chances of success of the project; 3. the need to define clear and more specific goals in order to make it easier to recruit volunteers for their delivery; 4. the need to collect data on people's personal assets in a systematic way in order for it to be usable (Giuntoli et al., 2012).

## Social and political action

If individuals remain at the small group level, the conditions leading to their sense of powerlessness would not be resolved. Equally, if individuals are compromised by being represented by others or engage in passive and indirect actions, for example, signing a petition, their level of influence will remain limited. Practitioners are involved in approaches in their day-to-day work in ways that can help their clients to become more critically aware and to take a more active role in collective action. This involves encouraging participation, partnership development and more direct actions, such as campaigns, civil protests and legal action.

Gaining control to influence economic, political, social and ideological change will inevitably involve individuals, groups and communities in a struggle with those already holding power. Within a programme context the role of the Practitioner is to build capacity and provide resources and technical support. But Practitioners also need to recognize that an empowering public health practice is a political activity and their role, at least in part, is to strive to challenge the dominant power-over discourse and practice. At some point, a community will recognize that there is the need to gain access to political influence and to resources at a broader level. This moves the community forward from engaging in a strategy of capacity building to one of empowerment (Laverack, 2007). Community empowerment and community capacity overlap as forms of social organization and mobilization that seek to address the inequalities in people's lives. Capacity building is the means by which an outcome of empowerment can be achieved through systematically building knowledge, skills and competencies. However, building community capacity is not isolated to a single outcome because the competencies that are developed can be transferable across social, political and economic issues.

In a programme context this can be in relation to particular issues around which clients act together to create, or to resist, change. The skills, competencies and capacities that they will need to develop can be supported as part of the everyday work of Practitioners. Finally, it is important to recognize that empowerment takes on meaning in relation to issues around which the group impetus grows or fades. There is therefore never absolute power or empowerment for individuals, groups and communities.

Social movements can provide an important way for people to achieve broader social and political change. They also provide a bridge between an ideology that many community-based organizations espouse on empowerment and liberation and the established discourse used in society.

# Health social movements

Although there is no real agreement as to the nature of social movements, they share a structure, a pattern of inter-relations and the formation of an identity that is recognized by its members. Formal social movements may possess bureaucratic procedures but they do not operate from within bureaucracies. Social movements exist within civil society and are developed by the people, often against systematic structures and ideologies held by those in authority (Pakulski, 1991). Health social movements (HSMs) strive for a transformation of values and for change rather than for a radical restructuring, to promote the health and well-being of others. HSMs are an important point of social interaction concerning the rights of people to access health services, personal experiences of illness and disability and health inequality based on race, class, gender and sexuality.

The growing awareness of health science that has become available through, for example, online media, has led to people challenging public health policy. This has been coupled with the negative publicity received about bio-medical abuses of authority, such as experimentation with contraceptives, radiation and immunization, that has created a heightened level of distrust among the public. People have discovered that collectively they can apply significant pressure to influence the policies that affect their health (Brown and Zavestoski, 2004). HSMs ultimately challenge state, institutional and other forms of authority to give the public more of a voice in policy and regulation.

HSMs overlap in their purpose and tactics but can be broadly categorized into three types (Brown et al., 2004):

1  Health access movements seek equitable access to health care services, for example, through national health care reforms and an extension of health insurance to non-insured sectors of the population.
2  Embodied health movements involve people who want to address personal experiences of disease, illness and disability by challenging of the scientific evidence and campaigning for medical recognition of their ideas or their own research. It can include people directly affected by a condition or those who feel they are an at risk group, for example, the HIV/AIDS movement.
3  Constituency-based health movements are concerned with health inequalities when the evidence shows an oversight or disproportionate outcome, such as the environmental rights movement.

HSMs are not the sole source of external influence on health policy but they can play an important role, one that is sometimes undervalued. Box 7.6 provides an example of the actions of one HSM, the environmental breast cancer movement, to influence policy on health care in the USA.

## Box 7.6 The environmental breast cancer movement

The environmental breast cancer movement in the USA was formed by a spill-over from the women's movement, AIDS activism and the environmental movements that created a HSM able to identify with those at risk from or affected by breast cancer. Maren Klawiter (2004, pp. 865–866) discusses the early experiences of women with breast cancer in the 1970s in the San Francisco Bay Area who endured isolation and

*(Continued)*

power inequalities structured around the doctor–patient relationship and gender. The breast cancer movement provided many people with the intellectual and emotional support they needed to be able to move forward collectively to address a personal issue. Using the lessons that they had brought with them they pressed for expanded clinical trials, compassionate access to new drugs and greater government funding. Twenty years later a new regime of breast cancer care had emerged influenced by the efforts of the environmental breast cancer movement. Women had access to feminist- and gay-friendly cancer centres, patient education workshops, support groups, a choice of medical alternatives and a role as part of the health care team that delivered the cancer treatment. Essentially, breast cancer care had become politicized and reframed as a feminist issue and an environmental disease.

HSMs have been effective in influencing others by changing individuals and the values that they hold through, for example, cognitive praxis and movement intellectuals. Cognitive praxis is the 'knowledge interests' that are held by a movement and the 'dynamic and mediating role that movements play in the shaping of knowledge' (Eyerman and Jamison, 1991, p. 47). This is the origin of new knowledge generated by a movement and 'intellectuals' within the movement draw upon and reinterpret established intellectual concepts. Cognitive praxis plays another important role, the development of new societal images and identities. Examples of how society transforms its self-identity through the knowledge generated by social movements include setting new problems for society to solve and advancing new values for ethical identification by individuals. The role of 'movement intellectuals' is to strategically plan and create new knowledge. As the movement matures and new organizations emerge, there may be a transformation in the relationship between the intellectuals and the movement. Movement intellectuals occupy the space created for them temporarily before they seek legitimacy elsewhere, for example, in academia, media and government agencies. They establish their new identities and thus act as a vehicle through which movement knowledge can be dispersed socially. In this way, intellectuals create movements and movements create intellectuals in processes within society to challenge conventional wisdom. Social movements can be the engines of social change and can create new knowledge and intellectuals that later become absorbed by society. Thus, they create a bridge between radical thinking and established knowledge constructions. In this way, the legitimization of the discourse on public health issues has been influenced through either the absorption of movement intel- lectuals into or their direct influence upon government, academic and other sector agencies (Eyerman and Jamison, 1991).

Public health itself is not a social movement because, while it may share an emancipa- tory discourse, in practice it is carried out within the controlling sphere of bureaucratic settings. Public health remains disease based, embracing a bio-medical interpretation of health and employing top-down approaches to programming driven by the reduction of morbidity and mortality.

Next, Chapter 8 takes the discussion of community empowerment further to exam- ine how Practitioners can work with marginalized and migrant populations and discusses the circumstances of Roma in Europe. The importance of resolving conflict in a programme context is also discussed.

# 8

# HELPING MIGRANT POPULATIONS TO BECOME EMPOWERED

## Introduction

The concepts of power and empowerment can hold different interpretations for people from different social and cultural backgrounds and who migrate to another country. Newly arrived migrants are often familiar with a different political context, and democracy and civil society may be new concepts. The newly arrived migrants may also not understand public health programmes that are designed to facilitate participation, needs assessment or critical awareness.

The differences in the interpretation of power and empowerment can include the degree of, or expectation of, control over the events in a person's life, the choices that they have, status within society and an understanding of how to access essential services. Contextual influences such as poverty (economic), social norms (socio-cultural), bureaucratic structures (political) and historical circumstances, can also lead to differences in their interpretation.

Laverack et al. (2007) undertook a study to determine the interpretation of power and empowerment in migrant Pacific peoples in Auckland, New Zealand. The predominant perception of power was of power-over an individual, group or community but also of how people could better themselves within society through taking advantage of educational opportunities. In a Pacific context, knowledge is power, and that power lies in the use of knowledge to advance one's understanding of the world. Power is gained when people are given the information or resources that will help them gain knowledge about issues that directly affect them, but does not mean that one person has to give up power in order for another to gain it. (A non-zero-sum interpretation of power is discussed in Chapter 2). Power can be shared between respective parties provided they have a 'voice' and are able to express their opinions. In migrant Pacific peoples in Auckland, the concept of empowerment was not based on an individual level of control but was built around a cultural framework of, for example, returning a favour, supporting other people's capacities and working as a family, group or community. The way in which people viewed their role differed from a westernized perception of individual action and the control over material resources to exert an influence.

Understanding the perceptions of migrants in regard to power and empowerment can have important implications for public health practice. There has been a tendency to combine migrants groups together under one ethnic category for the purposes of delivering health policy. Categorizing migrants under one homogeneous group runs the real risk of advantaging some at the expense of others; for example, in a competitive funding environment there should be equal opportunity to access resources. Equal opportunity should recognize the subtle cultural and organizational differences between groups and understand that accessing resources can sometimes be an unequal, zero-sum power situation. Laverack et al. (2007) found that that some Pacific peoples are socially and organizationally disadvantaged. Each Pacific population had their own strengths but also their own constraints on collectively organizing and mobilizing themselves to gain control of the limited resources available to improve their lives and health. Some Pacific peoples are better organized, have stronger leadership, more community participation and are better able to mobilize resources. Not surprisingly, these Pacific peoples are more successful at accessing resources such as government funding. Ideally, in a competitive public health environment there should be an equal opportunity for all communities to access funds, and therefore measures should be taken to ensure this happens during the process of allocating resources.

## Marginalization

Marginalization is a process by which an individual, group or community is denied access to, or positions of, power within a society (Marshall, 1998). Marginalization is relevant to public health because those people who exist on the fringes of a society can become excluded, for example, from access to essential services. It is a paradox of empowerment approaches that the marginalized are often unable to articulate their needs, are not represented or are not well informed and, as a result, do not have the opportunity to voice their concerns. The circumstances of their marginalization and the low self-esteem that this can produce can also contribute to mainstream public health programmes not involving them.

In practical terms, the marginalized are considered to be those who are most vulnerable, are not able to meet their own needs, have limited access to resources, are powerless or exist largely outside dominant economic, political, religious and social power structures. Marginalization can be based on gender, ethnicity, (dis)ability and sexual preference, and includes the elderly, people of a low socio-economic status and migrants. Marginalization should not be confused with the numerical value that can be placed on minority but instead should emphasize the social position of the group. The marginalized are subordinate segments of complex societies, have special physical or cultural traits and are held in low esteem by society. These traits bind their members, who share a conscious understanding of their circumstances (Simpson and Yinger, 1965). Marginalized people regard themselves as objects of collective discrimination, having been singled out for unequal treatment from the majority of others in the society in which they live.

Practitioners must have a clear understanding of the circumstances that cause the marginalization of their clients, for example, inequalities in access to services, stigma and negative societal attitudes that can exclude those who do not appear to conform to societal norms and values. Ideally, Practitioners work with those most in need and strive to avoid the establishment of a public health agenda that might exclude certain groups within society.

## Marginalization and migration

Migration, either in terms of internal migration where no national boundaries are crossed, or international migration where people move to another place across national boundaries, is an increasing challenge for public health. Migration is not always intended to be permanent and many people may wish to return to their home country at some stage in the future. For example, people may leave their home countries to look for better economic opportunities, because of oppressive political circumstances or conflict, to be with family or to seek an education. A significant factor in the evolution of how migration patterns have developed has been the advancements in the methods of travel (MacPherson and Gushulak, 2004).

Migrant communities can become socially and economically marginalized and Simpson and Yinger's (1965) interpretation used earlier of a feeling of belonging or not belonging has resonance for many migrants. Examples of migrants living as marginalized groups within society include ethnic minority groups (for example, Chinese or Turkish), religious groups (for example, Jewish or Muslim) and illegal or seasonal workers. Shifting labour markets have intensified migrant concentrations in urban areas and accelerated international migration to wealthier countries where there are better work opportunities. When living in a new country many migrants are faced with restricted legal rights, a poor understanding of the local language and culture, different religious beliefs and a lower socio-economic status. This can lead to feelings of exclusion and as a consequence migrants can be placed in a vulnerable position of poor physical and mental health that is compounded by a limited understanding of how to access health care and social services. Next, I discuss the link between migration and empowerment through a discussion of Roma in Europe, both as migrants and as established but marginalized residents.

## Roma migrants and empowerment

The Roma are the largest minority group in Europe with a population of 10–12 million people consisting of a variety of different ethnic groups. What these groups have in common is that they all face severe discrimination, racism and marginalization. 'Roma-phobia' has become a socially accepted feature in Europe in which the Roma have been labelled as a 'European problem' rather than as another minority group (van Baar, 2011, p. 204). Efforts to ensure Roma inclusion have been a priority in some countries; for example, in Sweden the welfare system provides for everyone such that they have equal social, political and economic rights. However, many Roma living in Sweden still face difficulties in gaining the same access to social, political and economic rights as non-Roma (Crondahl et al., 2015).

The number of Roma immigrants from Central East European countries into Western Europe has significantly increased since the political and economic changes of the 1990s and the transition of East Germany to a market economy. This led to mass unemployment and impoverishment in Central and Eastern Europe. Roma people experience discrimination everywhere but ethnic intolerance in a country does not appear to be the strongest push factor for migration. It is the high remuneration and generous welfare systems of Western societies that are the attraction, and it is in these societies that Roma more frequently find what they are looking for, in terms of paid labour. The preferred countries for Roma migration in Europe are Germany, the UK, Greece, Italy, Austria, Spain, Sweden and Switzerland. Other important factors for the choice of country are the nearness of the country, cultural similarities, the presence of migrant networks, better living conditions, advanced social and health care systems and a more stable political situation (Cherkezova and Tomova, 2013).

## Roma and participatory approaches

Participatory approaches can improve trust and enhance the inclusion of Roma perspectives within public health programmes (Kósa and Adany, 2007); for example, one study in western Sweden aimed to strengthen Roma empowerment, participation and a sense of community and to promote self-led social integration (Crondahl et al., 2015). The participatory approach was based on work integrated learning (WIL) and used three parallel tracks: (1) the continuation of basic education; (2) theoretical training; and (3) practical application of the training in real-life work. The approach included Roma education in issues related to community organizing, the social determinants of health and health promotion (Track 2). In parallel, the participants also worked in their local communities, practising and applying new knowledge and skills (Track 3) gained from the training. Roma in western Sweden place great importance on education and employment in regard to their health and well-being because of the need to self-manage their life situations, both at a collective and an individual level (Eklund-Karlsson et al., 2013). The combination of a participatory approach and WIL enhanced the participants' critical health literacy, and improved people's abilities to change health-related living conditions and their chances of empowerment by building on Roma needs. Through improved critical health literacy (see Chapter 6), the participants experienced greater control over their own lives and over social inclusion processes. WIL also helped to strengthen Roma identities and cultural awareness. This new insight strengthened the participants' skills, engagement and motivation for working for Roma rights and acted as a trigger for taking a more active role in their own communities. The study concluded that the use of health literacy and WIL as a participatory approach is an effective strategy for helping Roma people to enhance their own social inclusion (Crondahl and Karlsson, 2015).

## Roma empowerment

Working to help to empower Roma community-based organizations can be an effective strategy when focusing on three interrelated principles: community capacity building; a structured dialogue; and a simple funding mechanism. Good education and skills development are central to Roma empowerment but this should go beyond training to strengthen human resources and organizational structures, to improve leadership, governance and strategic planning. A structured dialogue with Roma community-based organizations helps to foster their involvement and this should always begin with a local needs assessment. National governments should also be encouraged to develop sub-granting financial mechanisms based on simplified procedures accompanied by strengthening partnerships with pro-Roma agencies and training in financial management (D'Agostino, 2014).

Central to a Roma perspective of empowerment is the desire to self-manage their life situations, at a collective and an individual level. Both a sense of power-from-within and power-over (see Chapter 2) are necessary for Roma to be able to enhance their participation, critical awareness and to improve people's health and well-being. Employment and income are two important aspects of the Roma sense of power-over. The labour market integration of the Roma has been poor and Roma are much less likely to have jobs than non-Roma or have jobs that earn much lower salaries than non-Roma (Cherkezova and Tomova, 2013). Equality is a UK-based support organization that aims to help empower Roma to resolve their expressed needs on employment, housing, education, health care and social welfare. The organization acts as a negotiator between Roma and the providers of services to help reduce social exclusion, discrimination and exploitation. In the UK, Roma have established communities in the north of England, East Midlands, Kent and north and east London, with an estimate of approximately 300,000 people, although many Roma avoid declaring their ethnicity and instead use their nationality. 'The Big Issue' is now one of the UK's leading social businesses and continues to offer homeless and vulnerably housed people the opportunity to earn a legitimate income. The company produces and distributes 'The Big Issue' magazine through a network of street vendors. Equality, with the support of 'The Big Issue', developed an empowerment project focusing on the employment of young Roma who were unemployed or seeking work. These Roma were offered literacy, numeracy and English language classes and 'into-work training', for example, in sales, customer service, budgeting and building self-confidence, to enhance their knowledge, skills and abilities to improve their chances of finding work. Participants also worked as the vendors of 'The Big Issue' magazine, buying each magazine upfront for £1 and selling it for £2, keeping the profit made for themselves and thereby earning some money while exploring other opportunities through the Equality Empowerment Project (Equality, 2015).

Social inclusion policy for Roma has focused on economic empowerment and has used approaches for job creation through a combination of socially sensitive investment and enhancing small entrepreneurial activity through microcredit. However, for Roma communities in Eastern Europe, microcredit has had a limited role in facilitating self-employment, primarily because Roma entrepreneurs generally lack financial support, are indebted and have been refused credit by banking institutions. One viable option is to facilitate Roma employment by focusing on the creation of sustainable jobs in the private sector (Open Society Foundations, 2012).

Box 8.1 provides a case study of how one town in Bulgaria was able to negotiate better working rights for Roma who had previously been forced to find work elsewhere, outside the country and under insecure terms and conditions.

## Box 8.1 Negotiating the working rights of Roma

In Kavarna, a town in north-eastern Bulgaria with a population of 11,549, the Roma are approximately 25% of the population and have 30% of children of school age. Only 6.1% of Roma in the municipality had a job, mostly under temporary employment. The Roma had tried to find work abroad, such as seasonal work as construction workers in Germany, Poland and Austria. However, the majority of Roma were forced to only work for three months, as this was the period of their visa in the EU for Bulgarian citizens. This resulted in many Roma finding work without permission and therefore earning less money and under harsher conditions. The mayor of Kavarna decided to negotiate an agreement in a number of Polish towns to allow Roma to work there legally, with registered companies and paying taxes. Incomes rose to over 3,000 Euro per month and the Roma were able to save to build houses in Kavarna, buy cars and to pay for the weddings of their sons. According to the mayor, the most important result of this change in the economic status of Roma was to help to reduce negative stereotypes towards them in Kavarna, and it was therefore a prerequisite for changing inter-ethnic relations in a positive direction (Tomova, 2013).

Roma place great importance on education in regard to their own health and well-being and that of their families. This is based on the need to have more power-over and to self-manage their life and health situations. Box 8.2 provides a case study of how authorities in Belgium have used school mediators to help Roma children by involving parents, as well as teachers, in decision making processes about their education.

---

### Box 8.2 Promoting education for Roma children through school mediators

In Belgium, education is compulsory for all children aged 6–18 years, including migrant children, and the regular attendance at school is a condition for parents to receive monthly welfare benefits. This policy aims to motivate parents in vulnerable families to be more involved in their children's education. The function of school mediators in Belgium is not to help children to learn, as this is the role of the teachers. School mediators visit migrant families when authorities feel that stricter supervision of parents is necessary or when a child has a problem, such as missing classes or academically under-performing. Their aim is to clarify the problem and involve parents in its solution. The school mediator aims to help parents to raise their aspirations and expectations about their own children, and to enhance the parents' responsibility for their children's school success. They help parents understand their rights, responsibilities and obligations towards their own children's school success. School mediators also provide teachers with information about Roma and their culture. They assist school staff in developing its intercultural policy and motivate teachers to reinforce Roma children's self-esteem. They also try to facilitate contacts between the teachers and Roma parents who have problems with language or show no interest in their children's education (Cherkezova and Tomova, 2013, p. 142).

---

## Helping migrant populations

Practitioners can play an important role in helping migrants by providing them with the knowledge, skills and resources that they require to address their needs. A major challenge for many Practitioners is to develop and maintain the trust of migrant communities. This is a long-term process of dialogue and commitment to encourage broader participation. The role of the Practitioner is to continue to listen and then to respond to migrant needs using a mix of strategies and appropriate channels of communication. One study, for example, found that an appropriate communication strategy for Chinese migrants included messaging in English, Mandarin and Cantonese distributed through a combination of channels of mass media, such as Chinese newspapers, Chinese TV and radio stations (Tse et al., 2011).

Migrants are more likely to be committed to the objectives of a public health programme if they have a sense of ownership in the issues being addressed. Top-down programmes in which the Practitioner directly controls what is happening can serve to reinforce a sense of subordination and dependency. Programmes that do not address migrant needs and that do not involve them in the process of assessment therefore have less chance of achieving their purpose. The first challenge is to identify the communities' own sources of power (resources, decision making authority, technical skills, local knowledge, etc.), rather than begin from the perspective that migrants are relatively powerless. The Practitioner looks for, and works from, areas in people's lives in which they are relatively powerful. For example, migrants may hold a great deal of authority in one aspect of their life, such as being a community leader, but possess very little authority in other aspects, for example, in the workplace, where they may have a low-paid job. Local leaders can be an important factor in enabling others to take control of the influences on their health and to help manage programmes once they have acquired the necessary competencies. Transferring responsibility is an ongoing process but over time, and as additional resources and skills are obtained, the community can take more control of the programme. This includes activities such as fundraising and liaison with other organizations that can be facilitated by having a systematic approach that aims to give more responsibility and involvement within the programme. However, the Practitioner's role is not to direct the community in how it should identify its own representatives. The community must decide who should and should not be their representatives. The Practitioner can help by ensuring all representatives have an equal opportunity to express their opinions in the management of the programme.

The second challenge is to assist migrants to create an adequate resource base for community action, and to do this the Practitioner can act as a link between external resources, such as government grants, and the migrant community. The use of flexible funding mechanisms is discussed in Chapter 10.

The third challenge is to assist the migrant community to resolve any internal conflict that may exist and it is this issue that I discuss next.

## Resolving conflict

Conflict can be a negative ingredient of the empowerment process as it takes attention away from important issues, divides communities and undermines individuals' power-from-within. However, if managed correctly, conflict can also be a positive ingredient. Dealing with conflict in a positive way can resolve disputes, help to release emotions and anxieties and make the community address sensitive issues, while at the same time improving co-operation and communication. The beginnings of conflict are often caused by poor communication, weak local leadership, struggles to gain access to limited resources and decision making, and the uncertainty of Practitioners about their role in how to resolve conflict (Laverack, 2009).

In Box 8.3 I provide an exercise that can help both Practitioners and clients to understand their own reactions in a position of power imbalance. In this exercise the power is represented by the allocation of resources. While the difference in allocation is minor, this is representative of more meaningful situations that can result in the participants making connections to other areas in their lives, where they may be unaware of the disparities of power (Coleman, 2000). The exercise can be used as part of a training activity for Practitioners or as a means of demonstrating to their clients the disruptive effect that conflict can have on a community.

---

### Box 8.3 Positions of power and resolving conflict

The trainers organize the space into two areas, each to accommodate half of the participants. One area is provided with markers, coloured pens, paints, coloured paper, scissors, magazines and other decorative items. In the other area there is one sheet of

*(Continued)*

blank paper and pencils. The participants are invited back into the room and randomly allocated to one of the two areas. The two groups are given the same objective: to develop a working definition of power. They are informed that once the groups have finished the exercise they will be asked to display their definitions, and a vote will be taken by everyone in the room to select the best and most attractive definition. The groups are then asked to begin the 30-minute exercise and the trainers actively support the group with the most resources, while actively ignoring the group with the least resources. The developed definitions are displayed and a discussion held about the best one, including the use of colour, attractiveness and technical content. The participants are also asked to discuss the dynamics of the two groups, their feelings and how they interacted during the exercise. Participants may be unaware of the disparities in resource allocation, may have tried to persuade the other group to give them extra resources or even to take resources without asking. These points are discussed in relation to the issue of power and conflict resolution. (Adapted from Coleman, 2000, pp. 127–128)

In conflict situations, those with the power-over tend to try to dominate and to offer few concessions and this can make it difficult to reach a negotiated agreement that is satisfactory to all parties. Those who are in a powerless position become alienated and are presented with two main options: (1) to resist by increasing their own resources, organization and mobilization and using this in tactics of disobedience; (2) to induce those with power to use it more benevolently and to be sympathetic to the inequality of those with less power (Coleman, 2000). To enable their clients to gain more power-over in (1) above or to be in a better position to negotiate in (2) above requires an approach to resolve conflict. These strategies can include providing training for conflict management, developing communication tools to better disseminate information, using listening to clarify understanding, providing a facilitated dialogue to map and resolve issues, and using approaches of critical awareness. These and other strategies are discussed in Chapters 4 and 6. Practitioners cannot be expected to do all of this in their everyday work but they can play an important role in helping to resolve conflict by simply assessing the situation, being a good listener and by ensuring full participation to clarify areas of conflict. An example of resolving cross-cultural differences is provided in Box 8.4 in the 'Resolving Differences-Building Communities Project' in the UK.

## Box 8.4 The 'Resolving Differences-Building Communities Project'

The 'Resolving Differences-Building Communities Project' started after conflict erupted between groups of Somalian and African-Caribbean youth in Leicester, UK. The Somalians were settled as new immigrants into poor socioe-conomic areas occupied by the African-Caribbean community, and this created inter-ethnic tensions. The Somalians found it difficult to assimilate into the British culture, had language constraints and could not easily access available services. The Project established a steering group made up of stakeholders from the two communities, with the task of

*(Continued)*

coordinating the management and implementation. The main purpose of the Project was to clarify the views and opinions of the two groups about one another through workshops and focus group discussions. Local people were trained and employed as cross-cultural facilitators to provide peer education, mediation and to recruit some 400 young volunteers. In particular, it was the role of the facilitators, assisted by Practitioners, that led to a reduction in prejudice, and they managed to directly avoid conflict because of their interaction and attempts to build cohesion (Laverack, 2009, p. 41).

Conflict resolution does not have to be a specialist area of work, especially when the issue of disagreement is not complicated. In practice, conflict can sometimes be resolved by simple clarification and discussion of the main concerns. This is a process that can be facilitated by a Practitioner using participatory approaches to promote discussion. In Box 8.5 I provide the example of one exercise that can be used by Practitioners to help resolve conflict: first, by mapping the main questions held between the different stakeholders involved and, second, by developing strategies to address each relevant concern.

## Box 8.5 Defining the issues of conflict

To carry out this exercise the Practitioner should have some prior knowledge about the key questions that will be asked and some of the solutions that can be discussed. This will help the Practitioner to focus the discussion on the practical and not on the personal points. The Practitioner should be able to first define the issues of the conflict in neutral terms that all participants can agree upon as follows:

1 The participants are asked to construct a list of key questions about the conflict and the potential solutions to the questions.
2 The participants and the Practitioner next identify sources of information regarding each of the key questions, for example, websites, local leaders, government officials, that are necessary to move into a problem-solving stage.
3 The participants are asked to prepare a summary of the conflict by comparing each question with a possible solution and a source of information. This can be usefully summarized in a table.
4 After a period of discussion between the different parties, the table can be rewritten to highlight how major changes in one conflict alter over time as circumstances change.

It is important to note that this type of a problem-solving exercise is merely a commitment to further analysis and discussion. (Adapted from Mitchell and Banks, 1998, p. 31)

Next, in Chapter 9, I discuss the means of collecting and analysing qualitative information as an important professional competence for the measurement of community empowerment. The measurement and visual representation of community empowerment are then discussed with examples of using the 'domains approach' and the spider web configuration in a public health programme.

# THE MEASUREMENT AND VISUAL REPRESENTATION OF COMMUNITY EMPOWERMENT

## Collecting and analysing qualitative information

The evaluation of empowerment approaches often use participatory techniques and qualitative methods, including one-to-one and focus group interviews that draw upon knowledge and experiences. In qualitative interviewing, the aim is to discover the interviewee's own framework of meanings and to avoid imposing the interviewer's assumptions. The interviewer needs to remain open to the possibility that the variables that emerge may be very different from those that might have been predicted at the outset. The interviewer needs to be sensitive to the language and concepts used by the interviewee and check that they have understood the respondent. The flexibility of the interviewing technique is that it can allow a change in the pace and direction of the interview to avoid any misunderstandings during the inquiry (Britten, 1995).

### Qualitative interviewing

Qualitative interviewing offers two main types that can be used for the evaluation of empowerment: unstructured and semi-structured. Unstructured interviews may cover only one or two issues and, while semi-structured interviews are also conducted using an informal structure consisting of open-ended questions that define the area to be explored, the interviewer may diverge in order to pursue an idea in more detail and depth. The less structured the interview, the less the questions are determined and standardized in advance of the interview. However, most interviews will have a list of core questions that define the areas to be covered. Questions should be open-ended, neutral, sensitive and clear to the interviewee, usually starting with questions that the interviewee can easily answer and then proceeding to more difficult and sensitive topics.

### Starting the inquiry to collect qualitative information

The initial part of the inquiry uses unstructured interviews with key informants to identify the main theme of empowerment in the specific cultural context. Unstructured one-to-one interviews are used to discover the interviewee's own framework of meanings. This type of interview dispenses with formal schedules and ordering of questions and relies on the social interaction between the interviewer and the informant to elicit information (Minichiello et al., 1990). The unstructured interview takes on the appearance of a normal everyday conversation. However, it is always a controlled conversation, which is geared to the interviewer's interests. The element of control is minimal but present in order to keep the informant 'relating to experiences and attitudes that are relevant to the problem' (Burgess, 1982, p. 107). More than one unstructured interview can be used so that further questioning can be based on previous interviews. These interviewers should consist mostly of clarification and probing for more detail. It is important to carry out as many unstructured interviews as are necessary to be sure that all the main headings for empowerment have been identified. Qualitative data should be collected until the interviewing reaches a point of 'data saturation', or when the interviewer is no longer recording new information. The point at which the interviewing is stopped is a contested issue but is flexible and is based on the discretion and experience of the interviewer (Mason, 2010). The interviewees can be different but the interviews are to be based on the same themes; for example, they might begin with the interviewer asking 'This interview is about empowerment in your cultural context. Can you tell me about your experiences, what you think this means and how it works in your community?' The interviews can be held at the interviewees' places of work, homes or in a neutral setting, at a predetermined and convenient time. The interviews are recorded either manually or by using a tape-recorder and normally last between 30 and 90 minutes.

## Gaining in-depth information

The findings of the unstructured interviews provide the main headings for the next part of the inquiry: semi-structured group interviews. The questions do not have a fixed order or wording, but act as a guide to the interviewer, who uses them in small groups consisting of participants of similar characteristics. The purpose of the interviews is to provide more depth and comprehension to the main headings and anecdotal information to highlight the findings. The selection of participants for the interviews is undertaken to ensure a representative range of age and socio-economic background of the people in the community.

Group interviews are a quick and convenient way to simultaneously collect data. This means that instead of the interviewer asking each person to respond to a question in turn, there is some interaction and people are encouraged to talk, ask questions, exchange anecdotes and comment on other experiences in the group. Some of the potential advantages are that the technique does not discriminate against people who cannot read or write and encourages participation and discussion, especially from those who might normally feel that they have nothing to say. However, the group setting may silence individual voices of disagreement and it is these contradictions that the interviewer may want to gain access to as part of the findings. The presence of other interviewees may also compromise the confidentiality of the session; however, groups are not always inhibiting and may actively facilitate the discussion of sensitive topics.

The success of the group interviews depends on both the skill of the facilitator and the discussion environment. Sessions should be relaxed and in a comfortable and familiar setting, refreshments may be available and the seating should be arranged in a sequence acceptable to the participants. The facilitator should be able to use the debate to continue the conversation beyond the stage where it might have otherwise ended and to encourage participants to elucidate their point of view and to clarify why they think as they do (Kitzinger, 1995).

## Keeping a record of the inquiry

A number of different notes can be used by the interviewer to help compile a record of events; for example, a notebook or laptop can be used to keep detailed records of events, conversations, activities and descriptions. The type of notes can be distinguished as either quick or fully comprehensive to record exactly what is said. Mental notes are made of discussions and observations, jotted notes are quick, and shorthand notes are used to remind the interviewer of events. Full field notes are the running notes made throughout the day, during or after the observational period, and are both descriptive and analytical. The descriptive notes portray the context in which the observations and discussions took place. The analytical notes try to make sense of what has been observed and may be made after the observation when the interviewer has more time to reflect and clarify his or her impressions (Glesne and Peshkin, 1992).

## Analysing the qualitative information

The aim of the analysis of the qualitative information is to look for both areas of common ground and differences between the respondents, rather than provide a number of separate accounts. There are software packages for qualitative data analysis, such as NVivo, which are designed for working with very rich, text-based information where deep levels of analysis, often on large volumes of data, are required. The recommended procedure for analysis in this approach uses a simpler, cut and paste technique, which is quick, simple and cost effective for small amounts of qualitative information. The field notes and transcribed interviews go through a process of disaggregation and reaggregation using the following steps:

1   The process of **disaggregation** begins when copies are made of the original field notes. The copies are used to identify a classification system for the major categories of discussion. The categories are identified by using colours to highlight their presence in the text. The recorded text is thoroughly reread and all the marked relevant phrases, sentences or exchanges of recorded conversation are checked.
2   Once the **colour coding** is complete the marked text is 'cut up' and sorted into files that have been marked, one for each category. The categories will form the headings of the discussion of the findings.
3   The process of **reaggregation** happens by re-reading each category file to analyse the content in its new context alongside information of a similar nature. New insights and confirmations begin to emerge and the structure of the findings and discussion begin to be formed.

## Facilitating the collection of qualitative information in a cross-cultural context

Public health programmes can involve different cultural groups. Before collecting qualitative information in a cross-cultural context there are issues which need to be taken into account. Being unfamiliar with a specific cultural context can make it more difficult for a Practitioner to reflect the reality of the situation and this means that important information might be lost. The most significant difficulties faced by Practitioners have been their inability to speak the local language, holding a different belief and value system, poor communication and different styles of interaction, attitudes towards time and political sensitivities. However, a knowledge of the local language, while important, is not essential, and building a rapport with potential clients is more essential, and is a function more of time spent on site and of interpersonal skills than it is of linguistics (Ginsberg, 1988).

In practice it may not be possible to have a facilitated group discussion because of the language and cultural differences between the Practitioner and clients. In this case, a facilitated design can be used that takes the cultural context into account. This requires a facilitator to be appointed to work with the Practitioner, one who is familiar with the cultural context. Facilitation introduces higher levels of control, the ability to focus on specific goals within a limited time period and is not merely translation or interpretation. Apart from accurate interpretation to the Practitioner during the course of the meeting, the ways in which facilitators work in the group setting, such as their role, style, background and appearance, are crucial in shaping interactions.

Figure 9.1 provides a typology of roles that a facilitator can play during any cross-cultural group meeting. Based on the levels of facilitator direction (leading and control techniques) and rapport (trust-building and distance-reducing techniques), four general types of role can be delineated: empathy; engagement; railroading; and disengagement (Laverack and Brown, 2003). Empathy involves the facilitator being able to achieve insightful understandings based on taking the point of view of the other. This is most likely when rapport (an equivalence of meaning construction between parties) is high and facilitator direction is low. Engagement also requires high rapport together with greater levels of facilitator direction, for example, where the facilitator encourages a particular direction for discussion. Low rapport results in role types that should be avoided. When rapport is lost or not gained, higher direction can force discussion to areas of lesser interest to the participants and is a kind of railroading. Low rapport combined with low levels of direction can leave the facilitator as a disengaged 'outsider' whose observations may lack validity. In practice, movement occurs between role types as the group meeting progresses, whereas the arrows in Figure 9.1 represent an ideal facilitation model with an interplay of engagement and empathy that characterizes the duration of the group meeting. High rapport is maintained and direction levels lowered and raised optimally according to the flow of the group interaction.

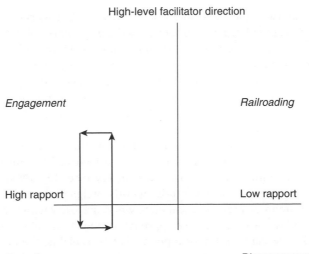

**Figure 9.1** Facilitator role types (Laverack and Brown, 2003, p. 4)

Laverack and Brown (2003) found that in a non-westernized context facilitators tended to do the following: they led the discussion and took a directive, rather than a participatory approach (railroading); they encouraged discussion but did not try to involve all the participants (loss of rapport); dominate and direct group interaction, and it was observed that they did not allow the focus of discussion to move towards the members as the workshop progressed (too directive); they left the room, and the participants were very able to continue each exercise but control of the discussion returned to the facilitators upon their return (too directive).

The requirement for good facilitation is crucial to many aspects of qualitative research. Cross-cultural facilitators are able to speak the local language, understand local customs and more easily explain complex concepts without the need for translation and this will help to expedite the meeting. Skilful facilitation is an issue common to qualitative approaches and the question 'how to ensure proper facilitation?' constantly needs to be addressed. This includes a successful balance between direction and rapport. Possessing the necessary skills and experience does not guarantee against facilitator bias, but proper training may reduce unintentional influences.

While high rapport is always the goal of skilful facilitation, in a cross-cultural context this may have to be achieved through roles embodying lower levels of rapport and differing levels of engagement. The purpose of this approach is to better position the facilitators to achieve an empathetic understanding of the participants. Cross-cultural contexts can provide essentially novel or unique issues and problems. The facilitators may have to be prepared to be more and less directive and engaged when collecting qualitative information, adapting their approach to the specific requirements of the participants. This can be described as an 'inward' and 'outward' movement by the facilitators towards a terrain of empathy conveying a similar pattern to those noted in qualitative and participant observatory research (Glesne and Peshkin, 1992).

## Using appropriate tools and the engagement of suitable personnel

In general, there are two other categories when working in a cross-cultural context that can be improved: the use of appropriate tools; and the engagement of suitable personnel. Appropriate tools for collecting cross-cultural information have been identified as a more naturalistic approach, for example, case studies and qualitative interviews which use the strong narrative and oral traditions of different cultures. Ideally, the approach should use both qualitative and quantitative information to cross-check the findings. The tools should also be flexible in terms of time and attitudes, be participatory and use culturally sensitive questions for data collection.

The skills and personal qualities required for suitable personnel to collect the cross-cultural information have been identified as: tolerance for ambiguity; patience; adaptiveness; capacity for tacit learning; and courtesy (Seefeldt, 1985). A number of authors have suggested that a team comprising both foreign personnel and a facilitator from the host community, preferably someone working closely with the public health programme, provides the most suitable approach (Chow et al., 1996). When it is not possible to work in a team, or if a local person is not available, then adequate training about the cultural context should be provided to anyone not from that specific cultural context (Russon, 1995). It is also important for the Practitioner to have a prior understanding of the fluid social dynamics and complex balance of relationships that occur between programme stakeholders in a cross-cultural context. Activities that may have little or no relevance to the Practitioner, such as the seating arrangements in a meeting, may have profound implications for the clients. This understanding can be improved through cross-cultural awareness training and better communication and listening skills (Cass et al., 2002).

## The measurement of community empowerment

The measurement of community empowerment has traditionally used qualitative information to provide dense descriptive accounts, based on the experiences of the participants, which produce a large quantity of data. This type of data can be difficult and time consuming for Practitioners to interpret. The trade-off is between the use of 'quick and dirty' data that is not in-depth, such as standardized checklists, compared to qualitative and sometimes long-term studies. The aim of an empowering approach is to provide all stakeholders with a role and a mutual understanding of the programme and to make Practitioners more sensitive to different needs within cultural contexts.

## The domains of community empowerment

Several authors have attempted to identify the areas of influence on community empowerment (Goodman et al., 1998; Laverack, 2001; Rifkin et al., 1988) and this has assisted in the identification of the social and organizational factors and is a step towards making evaluation more operational. The practical purpose is to provide a guide to Practitioners in their planning, application and evaluation of empowerment approaches in public health programmes. In particular, Laverack (2001) identified a set of nine 'domains' of community empowerment through a review of relevant literature, with particular reference to the fields of health, social sciences and education. The domains were categorized from a textual analysis of the literature and the validity of this data was cross-checked by other researchers. The nine domains of community empowerment were identified as follows:

1   Community participation;
2   Problem assessment capacities;
3   Local leadership;
4   Organizational structures;
5   Resource mobilization;
6   Links to other organizations and people;
7   Ability to 'ask why' (critical awareness);
8   Community control over programme management; and
9   An equitable relationship with outside agents.

A description of each domain is given in Table 9.1. The domains have proven to be robust across a range of settings and cultural contexts and have been successfully extended to provide a guide for the measurement of community empowerment in public health programmes.

Table 9.1   The empowerment domains (Laverack and Labonté, 2000)

| Domain | Description |
|---|---|
| Participation | Only by participating in small groups or larger organizations can individual community members act on issues of general concern to the broader community. |
| Leadership | Participation and leadership are closely connected. Leadership requires a strong participant base just as participation requires the direction and structure of strong leadership. |
| Organizational structures | Organizational structures in a community represent the ways in which people come together in order to socialize and to address their concerns and problems. |
| Problem assessment | Empowerment presumes that the identification of problems, solutions to the problems and actions to resolve the problems are carried out by the community. |
| Resource mobilization | The ability of the community to mobilize resources from within and the ability to negotiate resources from beyond itself is an important factor in its ability to achieve successes in its efforts. |
| 'Asking why' | This is the ability of the community to critically assess the causes of its own inequalities. |
| Links with others | Links with people and organizations, including partnerships, coalitions and voluntary alliances between the community and others, can assist the community in addressing its issues. |
| Role of the outside agents | The outside agent increasingly transforms power relationships such that the community assumes increasing programme authority. |
| Programme management | Programme management that empowers the community includes control by the primary stakeholders over decisions on planning, implementation, evaluation, finances, reporting and conflict resolution. |

I next discuss the implementation of the 'domains approach' and its potential as a participatory tool to build and measure community empowerment. The key question for Practitioners is: 'How has the programme, from its planning through its implementation, through its evaluation, intentionally sought to enhance community empowerment in each domain?'

## The domains approach

The domains approach provides a precise way to strengthen and measure community empowerment in a programme context, including a visual representation of the findings. The domains approach is used with communities, most often as a group of representatives, normally 10–15 people, in a facilitated workshop-type setting. The participants are first provided with five qualitative statements for each of the nine empowerment domains, written on a separate sheet of paper. The five statements for each domain are pre-ranked from 1 (the least empowering) to 5 (the most empowering) and these are provided in Table 9.2. The ranking is not shared with the participants during the implementation to avoid the introduction of subject bias. One study, for example, found that the sharing of pre-ranked statements with the participants

Table 9.2  The ranking for each empowerment statement

| Domain | 1. | 2. | 3. | 4. | 5. |
|---|---|---|---|---|---|
| **Community participation** | Not all community members and groups are participating in community activities and meetings, such as women, youth, men. | Community members are attending meetings but not involved in discussion and helping. | Community members are involved in discussions but not in decisions on planning and implementation. Limited to activities such as voluntary labour and financial donations. | Community members are involved in decisions on planning and implementation. Mechanism exists to share information between members. | Participation in decision making has been maintained. Community members are involved in activities outside the community. |
| **Problem assessment capacities** | No problem assessment undertaken by the community. | Community lacks skills and awareness to carry out an assessment. | Community has skills. Problems and priorities identified by the community. Did not involve participation of all sectors of the community. | Community identified problems, solutions and actions. Assessment used to strengthen community planning. | Community continues to identify and is the owner of problems, solutions and actions. |
| **Local leadership** | Some community organizations are without a leader. | Leaders exist for all community organizations. Some organizations are not functioning under their leaders. | Community organizations are functioning under leaders. Some organizations do not have the support of leaders outside the community. | Leaders are taking initiative with support from their organizations. Leaders require skills training. | Leaders are taking full initiative. Organizations are in full support. Leaders work with outside groups to gain resources. |

(*Continued*)

Table 9.2 (Continued)

| | | | | | |
|---|---|---|---|---|---|
| **Organizational structures** | Community has no organizational structures such as committees. | Organizations have been established by the community but are not active. | More than one organization which are active. Organizations have mechanism to allow their members to provide meaningful participation. | Many organizations have established links with each other within the community. | Organizations are actively involved in and outside the community. Community committed to its own and to other organizations. |
| **Resource mobilization** | Resources are not being mobilized by the community. | Only rich and influential people mobilize resources raised by the community. Community members are made to give resources. | Community has increasingly supplied resources, but no collective decision about distribution. Resources raised have had limited benefits. | Resources raised also used for activities outside the community. Discussion by community on distribution but not fairly distributed. | Considerable resources raised and community decide on distribution. Resources fairly distributed. |
| **Links to others** | None. | Community has informal links with other organizations and people. Does not have a well-defined purpose. | Community has agreed links but these are not involved in community activities and development. | Links are interdependent, defined and involved in community development. Based on mutual respect. | Links generating resources, finances and recruiting new members. Decisions resulting in improvements for the community. |
| **Ability to 'ask why'** | No group discussions held to ask 'why' about community issues. | Small group discussions are being held to ask 'why' about community issues and to challenge received wisdom. | Groups held to listen about community issues. These have the ability to reflect on assumptions underlying their ideas and actions. Are able to challenge received wisdom. | Dialogue between community groups to identify solutions, self-test and analyse. Some experience of testing solutions. | Community groups have the ability to self-test, analyse and improve their efforts over time. This is leading towards collective change. |

**Table 9.2** (*Continued*)

| Programme management | By agent. | By agent in discussion with community. | By community supervised by agent. Decision making mechanisms mutually agreed. Roles and responsibilities clearly defined. Community has not received skills training in programme management. | By community in planning, policy and evaluation with limited assistance from agent. Developing sense of community ownership. | Community self-manages, independent of agent. Management is accountable. |
|---|---|---|---|---|---|
| Relationship with outside agent | Agents in control of policy, finances, resources and evaluation of the programme. | Agents in control but discuss with community. No decision making by community. Agent acting on behalf of agency to produce outputs. | Agents and community make joint decisions. Role of agent mutually agreed. | Community makes decisions with support from agents. Agents facilitate change by training and support. | Agents facilitate change at request of community which makes the decisions. Agents act on behalf of the community to build capacity. |

unacceptably influenced their decisions. The participants progressively ranked themselves higher for each domain compared to when they had no prior knowledge of the ranking scale. The use of the ranking scales actually led to the introduction of subject bias such that the participants did not make an independent assessment but instead provided consistently high rankings to match the expectations of the facilitator and the other group members (Laverack, 1999).

The ranking of each qualitative statement allows the facilitator to give the assessment a quantitative value that can then be used to graphically plot the data. For example, for the domain 'Local leadership' the ranking statements and numbers are provided below. If the participants choose the statement 'Some community organizations are without a leader', this domain will be plotted, for example in a spider web configuration, with a rating of 1.

**Table 9.3**   Example of statements for local leadership

| Domain | 1 | 2 | 3 | 4 | 5 |
|---|---|---|---|---|---|
| **Local leadership** | Some community organizations are without a leader. | Leaders exist for all community organizations. Some organizations not functioning are under their leaders. | Community organizations are functioning under leaders. Some organizations do not have the support of leaders outside the community. | Leaders are taking initiative with support from their organizations. Leaders require skills training. | Leaders are taking full initiative. Organizations are in full support. Leaders work with outside groups to gain resources. |

Taking one domain at a time, the participants are asked to select the statement that most closely describes the present situation in their community. The statements are not numbered or marked in any way and each is read out loud to encourage group discussion. The selection of a statement by the participants is then based on their own experiences and knowledge.

Next, it is important that the participants record the reasons that justify their selection of a particular statement for each domain. This will assist later participants, who make subsequent measurements and will need to take the previous record into account. It also provides empirically, observable criteria for the selection. This overcomes one of the weaknesses in the use of qualitative statements, that of reliability over time or across different participants making the assessment (Uphoff, 1991). The justification needs to include verifiable examples of the actual experiences of the participants taken from their community to illustrate in more detail the reasoning behind the selection of the statement. For example, taking the statement used above, 'Some community organizations are without a leader', the justification could be that local leaders have not yet been elected or that a disagreement between leaders has delayed a decision about who should be attending community meetings.

The sum of the measurement is a set of nine qualitative statements, one for each domain, which represent the strengths and weaknesses of empowerment in the community, at that particular time. The measurement, analysis and interpretation of this information should be shared with everyone, including policy makers as well as the community members. The information may also have to be compared over a specific time frame and between the different components of a programme. For this purpose, a visual representation of the measurement of each domain is a useful way to interpret and share the information in a programme context.

## The visual representation of the measurement

Several authors have used visual representations to measure community-based approaches; for example, John Roughan (1986), a community development practitioner, devised a wheel configuration and rating scales to measure personal growth, material growth and social growth for village development. The rating scale had ten points that radiated outwards like the spokes of a wheel for each indicator. Each scale was plotted following an evaluation by the village members to provide a visual representation of growth and development. However, the approach used 18 complex, interrelated indicators, such as equity and solidarity, to measure village development. Rifkin et al. (1988) in Nepal and later Bjaras et al. (1991) in Sweden used a simpler approach of five factors: leadership; needs evaluation; management; organization; and resource mobilization. The approach was not carried out as a self-evaluation by the community and essentially did not include strategic planning; however, these early experiences have provided the basis for subsequent practical tools for visual representation, including the spider web configuration.

## The spider web configuration

The spider web configuration is used to graphically plot the rankings of a measurement and has been successfully applied to community empowerment for visual representation in public health programmes. The spider web configuration is specifically designed to be used with the domains approach, as discussed earlier in this chapter, and uses readily available computer spreadsheet packages. The spider web configuration is inserted from the chart wizard using a standard radar chart with markers and then there is a series of simple steps to set the data range, the chart options and the chart location. The quantitative rankings from the measurement can be plotted and used to compare changes in the same community, between different communities and over a specific time frame. The spider web provides a quick picture of the strengths and weaknesses within a community and between communities in the same programme. The community members and the outside agent can provide a textual analysis to accompany the visual representation to explain why some domains are strong and others are not. The visual and textual analysis can then be used to better inform the development of strategies to build community empowerment during a specific time period, such as between programme reporting cycles.

### Experiences of applying the spider web configuration

The spider web in Figure 9.2 shows a distribution of high and low ratings of eight domains for Kowanyama, an Aboriginal community in Far North Queensland, Australia. In general, the measurement of the domains was quite low, as the Health Action Team that carried out the measurement using a domains approach was in the early stages of development. Participation was ranked the highest as the members reported active involvement in monthly meetings. The need to obtain support from leaders outside the Health Action Team and being recognized by the wider community as the lead local health advisory group was identified as a key strategy, including a range of marketing and promotional activities. Training was another strategy identified by the Health Action Team to develop skills in specific areas, including resource generation, as well as a Memorandum of Understanding with the local Shire Council (Laverack et al., 2009).

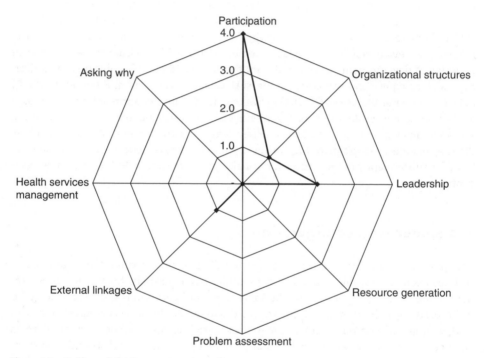

**Figure 9.2**   Spider web for Kowanyama, Australia

The spider web in Figure 9.3 provides an example of two measurements, taken in the same community, Ak-Terek in Kyrgyzstan (Laverack, 2007, p. 97), made six months apart. The community's assessment showed that it had made progress, with the support of the programme, in strengthening all the domains with the exception of critical assessment. The programme had initially carried out a needs assessment; however, the community recognized that empowerment had to go further than this to critically examine the broader (social, political, economic) causes of their powerlessness. This is a crucial stage towards developing appropriate strategies and demonstrates the ability of the community to look outwards and to think contextually rather than continuing to focus on internal or local issues. Strategies such as photo-voice (see Chapter 6) have been developed to strengthen the critical awareness of a community and can be used as an approach in public health programmes.

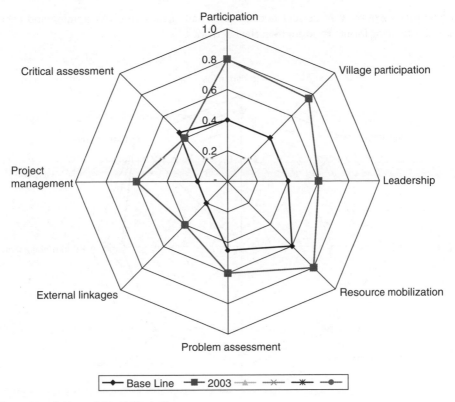

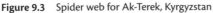

**Figure 9.3**  Spider web for Ak-Terek, Kyrgyzstan

Programmes in which there are more than one community intervention can also make a baseline for empowerment as an average value for each domain of each measurement. The measurement of community empowerment is compared with an average value baseline taken from the other measurements in the programme to give a comparison across the nine domains. In this way, the progress of any particular community in building empowerment can be assessed against other activities in other communities in the same programme.

The spider web configuration can also be used to cross-check an assessment made by the community. If the measurement of each domain is considered to be too high, for example, the outside agent, in collaboration with the community, can undertake an independent assessment of the findings. Figure 9.4 provides an example of an assessment made by two women's groups in Nepal, using a spider web configuration to provide a visual representation (Gibbon et al., 2002). This assessment used a ten-point rating scale. The spider web was plotted by hand on newsprint by the co-worker and representatives from two women's groups, who found the information it provided helpful for comparing changes over time and important for discussing why they had given slightly different assessments for the same domain. However, the co-worker felt that the overall assessment was too high and so carried out her own independent assessment based on her knowledge of the community. It confirmed that the high ratings for each domain that were made by the women's groups were correct because they had already received training and other capacity-building inputs to strengthen their activities.

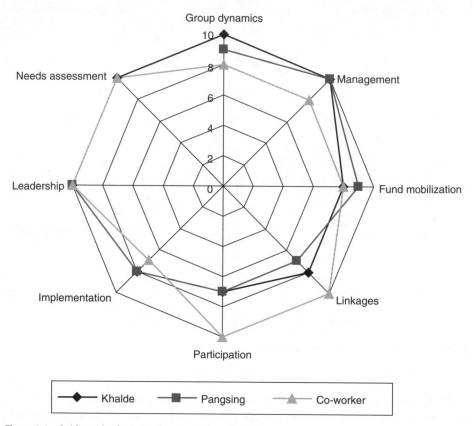

**Figure 9.4** Spider web of a co-worker assessment, Nepal

Next, in Chapter 10, I discuss what the future of public health programming will have to look like in order to be more successful in achieving empowerment goals. To do this, public health will have to find better ways of engaging with communities to share their priorities and to include them as an asset in the programme, to systematically build their capacity, develop more flexible funding mechanisms and be creative in scaling-up successful local initiatives.

# 10

# PUBLIC HEALTH, POWER AND EMPOWERMENT

In this book I have argued that power and empowerment are central to public health. I have also argued that Practitioners are faced with constraints when trying to use a more empowering approach in their work. In the final chapter, I discuss where we presently are in practice and what public health will have to look like in order to be more successful in achieving empowerment goals in the future.

## Why we are where we are

Public health programmes have been predominately professionally driven, top-down, pre-packaged and with a bio-medical focus. It has been the Practitioner who has exerted control over the programme through its implementation, management and evaluation (Laverack, 2007). The top-down approach has used epidemiological data to address population-based issues, including the increase in obesity, cancers and dangerous consumptions (Wanless, 2003). The dominance of this approach has meant that Practitioners have found it difficult to use empowerment approaches in their everyday work (Loss and Wise, 2007). Empowerment or bottom-up approaches assist the community to identify its own needs and to communicate these to the top structures of programme design and policy development. Needs assessment can be an important first step for Practitioners to engage with communities and to begin the process of empowerment. The role of the Practitioner is to enable their clients to identify actions to address their needs by providing technical support and resources and by building community capacity. The two agendas (top-down and bottom-up) do not always share the same goals and this can create a 'top-down versus bottom-up tension' in a programme context. Top-down public health agendas are typically centred on improving health through, for example, promoting healthy lifestyles, physical activity and a modification of diet. The lifestyle agenda has proved attractive to many political leaders because it promised easily quantifiable and achievable results within a short time frame, dealt with high-prevalence health problems, such as obesity, was simple (Gangolli et al., 2005) and offered powerful future cost savings in health care services for people suffering from chronic diseases (Bernier, 2007). The lifestyle agenda has also shifted the focus away from awkward political decisions that underlie poor health rooted in poverty and inequality (Labonté and Laverack, 2008).

Many top-down programmes have had only modest success and mostly with higher socio-economic groups. In Australia, for example, between 1998 and 2004 there was a 9% decrease in smoking in the lowest quintile compared to a 35% decrease in the highest quintile (Baum, 2007). In Canada, over the period 2000–2005, a top-down programme to increase physical activity in urban and rural communities found that 30% of people had become more active while 14% had become less active. Significantly, the change in physical activity had occurred in the higher socio-economic groups with little or no effect on low socio-economic groups, adolescents, ethnic minorities or indigenous people (Saskatoon Regional Health Authority, 2005). These trends have led some commentators to suggest that top-down programming may have had no effect in closing the gap between the healthy wealthy and low socio-economic groups. It may even, at least temporarily, have led to an increase in inequalities in health (Baum, 2007; Nutbeam, 2000). In certain circumstances this may have been made worse by public sector cuts that reduced health prevention and promotion services to the poor or by weakened safeguards on harmful goods, such as access to and advertising of junk food. The ability of the wealthy to afford the many health services and products offered by the private sector may have also been largely inaccessible to low socio-economic groups.

Top-down programming has relied heavily on strategies of the behavioural sciences and has largely employed health education modelling to raise awareness levels and to bring about individual behaviour change. Health education messaging has in some cases remained unchanged for many decades, for example, in regard to daily physical exercise and nutrition (Nutbeam, 2000). The modest success achieved through top-down public health programming has not therefore been a result of the issues it chooses to address or the messages it chooses to communicate. It has been because of the way in which public health programmes have been delivered. Top-down programming has relied heavily on strategies that have failed to engage with marginalized people and on ineffective communication interventions. Low participation in and motivation for top-down goals have hindered its progress to achieve the goal of closing the gap in health status between different social and economic groups in society.

## Giving communities a stronger role in public health

Practitioners, and the agencies that employ them, are increasingly recognizing the value of involving communities in the planning and decision making processes of public health programmes. These collaborative partnerships seek to address the agendas of both the community and outside agencies in a manner that suits both parties and recognizes local expertise and existing social connections. One project that has been successful in combining both top-down and bottom-up approaches is the 'like minds, like mine' project, which aimed to counter stigma and discrimination associated with mental illness in New Zealand. This project evolved by using a combination of top-down mass media and community education, by building community leadership and participation and by developing an infrastructure that used culturally specific approaches (Ministry of Health, 2003).

However, in practice communities are not regularly involved in decision making in public health programmes beyond initial consultation processes. This can leave communities feeling alienated from the changes taking place as a result of the programme and the impact it has on their lives. The contribution that communities can make in meeting health goals has also not received sufficient attention within public health programmes. The emphasis has been on collecting evidence at a population level and on working through health sector organizations to deliver interventions supported by professionals. Governments have placed an emphasis on professionally led interventions to improve health rather than on solutions designed and delivered by the communities themselves. At best this has failed to mitigate the effect of inequalities and at worst it may have contributed to the unfair distribution of resources within society (South et al., 2013).

To be more successful in the future in giving communities a stronger role and in achieving empowerment goals, public health will have to consider the following issues:

1  Engage communities to share their priorities;
2  Build community capacity;
3  Use mechanisms for flexible funding;
4  Build on successful local initiatives; and
5  Provide the means to allow community feedback.

## Engage communities to share their priorities

A major step to improving public health in the future will be to better accommodate top-down and bottom-up agendas. The key to this is for Practitioners to engage with communities during the planning stage to identify their needs and then to incorporate these within the design of the programme (see Chapter 3). Engaging with people in a programme context is crucial but it is not straightforward; for example, research in the UK has shown that of 80% of people who claimed to want to get involved in public services, when further questioned only 25% were actually prepared to give up their time (Confederation of British Industry, 2006). In the future, public health will be more successful if it can maintain a high level of participation and motivation among the programme participants. Box 10.1 provides an example of the type of pattern of the low level of participation in society.

---

**Box 10.1 Patterns of participation**

There is evidence to suggest that some people are reluctant to engage in more direct forms of participation; for example, in New Zealand one study showed that of the 89% of respondents to a petition only 19% attended a demonstration, 17% joined a boycott, 4% joined in a strike and only 1% were willing to take action (Perry and Webster, 1999) to try to influence a policy issue. This is a particular pattern with young people, members of ethnic minorities and those in low socio-economic groups, who are the least likely to be involved (Hayward, 2006). And yet, marginalized groups are the most likely to be affected by policy decisions because they have less of an economic buffer to protect them from changes in, for example, opportunities for employment and in changes to welfare policies.

---

Engaging with people is especially important when working with minorities, indigenous and low socio-economic groups who can become marginalized, as I discussed in Chapter 8. The engagement process can be based on a need that has already been identified by the community in order to provide a point of mutual interest around which the programme can develop. Box 10.2 provides an example of engaging a community to take responsibility on some of the tough questions in regard to a local road maintenance project.

**Box 10.2 Improving local involvement in road maintenance**

A private company was asked by Oxfordshire County Council to develop a solution to increase the life of a major road in Oxford, UK, including junctions, access and traffic calming. The work was planned to interfere as little as possible with local businesses and residents, by avoiding busy seasons and working when premises were closed. Road-user groups, local businesses and the police were involved from the design phase through regular public meetings. Residents were asked to choose from a series of options for the difficult decisions, such as when to work at busy junctions. The work itself was broken down into sections covering 200m of road, and residents were told dates in advance and businesses were allowed to continue deliveries. The road maintenance was planned around the convenience of local residents and businesses who were also involved in making decisions on an ongoing basis. This was formalized as a 'neighbourhood charter' or a two-way partnership between communities and a service provider, such as a construction contractor. The partnership helped to ensure that the work started and finished on time by helping to identify problems in advance, and resulted in a higher level of local participation and client satisfaction. Other projects have employed a Watchman-in-Chief who engages with businesses, service users, parish councils, the Highways Agency and local representatives. Other watchmen identify issues across the area and feed back to the Watchman-in-Chief. The Watchman role provides a non-bureaucratic, informal method through which the outside agency can keep in touch with a range of stakeholders when appropriate, enabling feedback and communication. The information provided is realistic and accurate and always allows local residents to provide their opinions and, if necessary, to be involved with the decision making processes (Confederation of British Industry, 2006).

Accepting the expertise offered by local people and sharing professional expertise so that the members can build their own empowering capacities can be difficult for some Practitioners. The aim is to facilitate the sharing of power in a way that involves the provision of both services and resources, at the request of the community, in a culturally and socially acceptable manner. This is power-with, discussed in Chapter 2. However, there have been few large-scale, well-resourced programmes that have systematically involved communities (South et al., 2013). The reasons for this are varied but the perception that communities lack the knowledge and skills to solve their problems, a lack of trust between government and civil society and an unequal distribution of control over decision making (being largely from the top-down) have contributed to this situation.

## Voluntary work

Voluntary work or lay health work can be an important way for people to participate in public health programmes, although it poses the challenge of how to effectively utilize the volunteers in a meaningful way. High volunteer turnover rates and the need for regular training, multiple incentives and the monitoring of duties mean that volunteerism is not necessarily a cheap or easy option for public health programmes.

Volunteerism is an activity that involves spending time doing something for free that aims to benefit the environment or other people, including close relatives (Volunteering

England, 2012). Volunteerism is an important aspect of public health work but is different to the voluntary sector, which provides an infrastructure for involvement across all not-for-profit organizations, voluntary, community, charity and social associations.

Volunteers are sometimes trained in the areas that they work, such as education and counselling, while others provide services on an as-needed basis, such as outreach, home visiting and community kitchens. The Cardio-vascular Health Awareness Programme (CHAP) in Ontario, Canada, for example, recruits local volunteers to help carry out health checks, such as measuring blood pressure. People at risk can then be referred to a doctor, helping to reduce the workload of other health professionals who would normally have to undertake this type of routine work (South et al., 2013).

Lay health workers are members of the communities where they work, selected by their communities, answerable to their communities for their activities, supported by the health system but not necessarily part of its organization (World Health Organization, 2007b). Lay health workers are without clinical training and undertake basic health care and preventive work. They have been an effective means to engage communities in public health programmes by actively involving people in peer support, as opinion leaders and to act as a bridge between communities and health services (South et al., 2013). Volunteers can provide a valuable network of local contacts and many community-based organizations depend on the efforts of volunteers who, behind the scenes, work tirelessly doing day-to-day activities (Winfield, 2013). Volunteers usually receive no pay, although their role can be fulfilling and can bring many benefits to the volunteer, such as improving self-confidence and skills. Volunteering should not cost the volunteer, that is to say that volunteers should be reimbursed financially for costs incurred, for example, travel, accommodation and food. One of the most critical problems for volunteerism is the high rate of attrition that can lead to a lack of programme continuity, volunteer burn-out and an increase in costs and in time to train new volunteers.

Volunteers can become dissatisfied with not receiving any incentives to carry out the services that they provide and lose their motivation to work. If this situation continues it can have a negative effect on the programme outcomes and on the role of other volunteers.

An international review (Bhattacharya et al., 2001) of community workers found that successful projects had multiple incentives over time to provide more job satisfaction. Incentives do not have to be monetary but could be in-kind, such as clothing or an appreciation of the role of volunteers through greater professional support. The review concluded that the sustainability of voluntary inputs into health programmes depends on several key factors, including the following:

▶ Volunteers should maintain a transparent relationship with the community such that they remain accountable to its members for their activities.
▶ The programme should plan for a high turnover of volunteers, for example, by having shorter but more regular training.
▶ Volunteers should continue to be made to feel valued by the health system by collaborating with other health professionals, for example, in outreach activities.
▶ The spirit of volunteerism should be maintained for as long as possible and when incentives are introduced these should be multiple and matched to duties and responsibilities.
▶ Regular monitoring of duties should always provide feedback to the volunteers about their performance.

## Build community capacity

An empowering public health programme must have a clearly defined strategy of how it will build community capacity from planning, through implementation and management, to evaluation. Community capacity is achieved through systematically building knowledge, skills and competencies at a local level. Without this focus the community can become dependent on an outside agency to provide support and resources without its members themselves taking greater control. Capacity building includes two key areas:

1 The capacity of the community is strengthened so that members can better define, assess, analyse and act on health (or any other) needs. This involves the development of specific skills, which contribute to their overall capacity. These skills may be used later to sustain the programme outputs or to address a variety of other circumstances. Capacity building therefore has a generic characteristic that is not limited to addressing only one issue.

2 The capacity of the community to take more control of the programme is enhanced. This involves skills development, for example, in management, budgeting, report writing, needs assessment and participatory evaluation. These are skills that the community can also use when it is involved in managing other programmes.

Interest in community capacity building as a strategy for sustainable skills, resource mobilization and participation in public health has developed because of the requirement to prolong programme gains (Gibbon et al., 2002). Community empowerment and community capacity overlap closely as forms of social organization and mobilization that seek to redress the inequalities in people's lives (Laverack, 2007). The capacity building process can be systematically strengthened through public health programmes by using a 'domains approach'.

## Use mechanisms for flexible funding

Capacity building often involves the provision of resources to support local initiatives. To meet this demand the outside agent should be flexible in the type and timing of resources that they are prepared to provide to support the community. In a programme context resources are often designated to a specific budget category, for example, health education or screening services, which may not meet the resources requested for community initiatives, for example, the costs to hold a community meeting. These activities may be difficult to justify as being directly relevant to public health but they nonetheless build the social dimension of communities by fostering a sense of belonging, connectedness and personal relationships. Funding bodies must therefore be able to think outside the 'health box' to develop suitable prototypes for financial support, for example, for matching counterpart contributions and for covering recurrent community costs (Commonwealth of Australia, 2000). Actual examples of how health funding bodies have used resources to support locally based initiatives include school and community gardens in Canada, the safer parks scheme in New Zealand, walking school buses in Australia, virtual communities in the USA and the green gyms and allotment junkies in the UK (Centre for Disease Control and Prevention, 2006).

Funding agencies can be reluctant to take risks with resources for programme activities which they feel are unpredictable or that cannot be measured. Funding small-scale initiatives can be a useful way to determine the validity of a programme design with a view to expand on successful community outcomes. Joan Wharf-Higgins et al. (2007) in British Columbia, Canada, looked at 12 regional seed-funded (short-term grants up to $4,500 Canadian) initiatives for chronic disease prevention. They found that those initiatives with most capacity building had a better chance of success, especially if resources could be found for the longer term as seed funding was too short-term to allow organic growth of the organization. The conclusion was that 10 out of the 11 initiatives continued beyond the funded period and that partnerships between communities and government agencies can work towards achieving sustainability.

In 2013 the Health Promotion Agency of New Zealand began delivering the Active Healthy Strong Community Partnership Programme aimed at improving nutrition and increasing physical activity. The programme provided up to $5,000 NZD to support community groups and organizations to develop and implement initiatives that provided opportunities for families to be physically active together. The programme targeted families with children under five years and had a focus on Māori, Pacific Island and low-income families. A second priority group was pregnant and breastfeeding women, and women with children under five years, again with a focus on Māori, Pacific Island and low-income families. Evaluation results indicate that 14 of the 18 projects achieved above the expected level of outcome, often driven by good participation rates. The micro-grants supported both tangible outcomes, stimulated by at least short-term community participation, and helped to maintain, and in some cases extend, community networks (Health Promotion Agency New Zealand, 2015).

## Build on successful local initiatives

A key turning point in the empowerment of a community is when it begins to address issues that go beyond local needs. Through the support offered by the programme, the local priority develops into an understanding of the underlying causes of the lack of control in people's lives, for example, how used syringes in a public park are a symptom of poor policing and anti-social behaviour in the neighbourhood. Programme support can then lead to broader social and political actions, for example, lobbying for better local policing and a policy on cleaning and monitoring public parks. This action has a better chance of success if funding bodies are willing to be creative to scale-up local initiatives and to allow bottom-up approaches to develop within top-down programming.

### Scaling-up local initiatives

Scaling-up remains an important unresolved question in many public health programmes: Are governments able to scale-up in partnership with community-based organizations to ensure benefits at a population level? Obviously, this requires the right level of political commitment, but examples of how scaling-up has been achieved include partnerships such as the Bangladesh Rural Advancement Committee and the Grameen Bank. Women in Bangladeshi communities became more empowered through micro-financing with the help of the Grameen Bank. The small loans were intended to give women more control over decisions regarding income generation and health. The success of the outcomes and loan repayments was attributed to the solidarity of community organizations, social support and the financial advantage offered by the loan (Papa et al., 2006).

While there is no real agreement on the level of increase that a programme has to reach to become 'scaled-up', it is usually considered to be the coverage of benefits to as many people within a specified area as possible, more quickly, more equitably and more sustainably (CORE Group, 2005). The problem begins when pilot projects are not planned to be scaled-up even when successful and are initially delivered as high-cost and low-participant activities. Scaling–up requires a planned process to be in place to expand on successful local initiatives once they have been tested, for example, by adding a creative initiative to an existing larger top-down programme.

Programme experiences of scaling-up have shown that certain principles apply when expanding on creative local initiatives and include: test and evaluate an initiative to determine its successfulness and feasibility to go to scale; include all stakeholders from the beginning; scale-up with broader policy; and promote equity and equality. Whether working with existing groups or new ones, in a partnership or directly engaging with the community, the roles and responsibilities of those who facilitate the 'scaling-up' process must be clearly defined. Small-scale projects are often successful because they are structured in such a way as to accommodate local power relationships. Scaling-up can result in these power dynamics becoming disrupted and roles at a local level not being acknowledged in a meaningful way. The impact, intentional or not, can then have an effect on the scaling-up process, for example, through a lack of participation and lower community contributions (Earle et al., 2004).

Expanding on successful local initiatives is important to gain greater and more equitable benefits but this process must be sensitive to the issue of power dynamics at all levels. It is therefore important to ensure that community feedback is received during the programme to identify any potential constraints for success.

## Provide the means to allow community feedback

The evaluation of public health programmes should address the concerns of all the stakeholders and provide information about its impact, operation, progress and achievements. Funding agencies will want to see value for money, Practitioners will want to see improvements in health and communities will want to see their needs being addressed.

In top-down programming, evaluation can be used as an instrument of control through performance measurement of targets by monitoring the operational elements of the implementation. The evaluation typically uses predetermined indicators, towards which the community members do not contribute, and is often implemented by an agency. In this approach there are few mechanisms that allow communities to have a voice or to provide feedback about how they have assessed the programme.

Bottom-up programming places the focus on participatory self-evaluation and away from conventional expert driven approaches. This means a fundamental shift in the power relationship between the Practitioner and the beneficiaries of the programme, one in which the control over decisions is more equitably distributed. An evaluation that empowers ensures that it addresses local concerns and has the means to allow communities to provide feedback. In turn, this information allows Practitioners to make informed decisions, even beyond the programme goals. Evaluation that empowers emphasizes people being actively involved in the evaluation process. The evaluation itself then becomes an empowering experience by building the capacity of the participants. In the future public health may have to reach a compromise between top-down and bottom-up styles of evaluation to allow communities to play a more active role.

The spirit in which this book has been written is for Practitioners to purposefully share power-with their clients and not to use it as a means to gain power-over them. The extent to which this happens will depend on how far Practitioners are willing to relinquish control in their everyday work and how honest Practitioners are prepared to be about their role in achieving an empowering practice. Given the constraints faced by many Practitioners, this can be a challenge. In this book, I explain how public health agencies, and the Practitioners that they employ, can use strategies to overcome this challenge and to make their work more empowering. The book offers a gradual way forward to develop public health rather than calling for a radical reorientation of practice. The way forward is more empowering for both Practitioners and their clients, who will find the creative ways that are provided in this book a motivation to enable others and to work together in a way that shares power and leads to a better public health practice.

# REFERENCES

Accident Compensation Corporation (2006) Entitlement claims to ACC from July 2004-June 2005. Statistics for Asian ethnic groups. Accident Compensation Corporation, Auckland, New Zealand.

Allmark, P. and Tod, A. (2006) How should public health professionals engage with lay epidemiology? *Journal of Medical Ethics*, 32: 460–463.

Allsop, J., Jones, K. and Baggott, R. (2004) Health consumer groups in the UK: A new social movement. *Sociology of Health & Illness*, 26(6): 737–756.

Anderson, E., Shepard, M. and Salisbury, C. (2006) 'Taking off the suit': Engaging the community in primary health care decision-making. *Health Expectations*, 9: 70–80.

Antonovsky, A. (1979) *Health, Stress and Coping*. San Francisco, CA: Jossey-Bass Publishers.

Appadurai, A. (2004) The capacity to aspire: Culture and the terms of recognition. In Rao, V. and Walton, M. (eds) *Culture and Public Action*. Stanford, CA: Stanford University Press, Chapter 3.

Baggott, R. (2000) *Public Health: Policy and Politics*. London: St. Martin's Press.

Barnes, M. and Gell, C. (2011) The Nottingham Advocacy Group: A short history. In Barnes, M. and Cotterell, P. (eds) *Critical Perspectives on User Involvement*. University of Bristol, UK: Policy Press, Chapter 2.

Bassett, S. F. and Prapavessis, H. (2007) Home-based physical therapy intervention with adherence-enhancing strategies versus clinic based management for patients with ankle sprains. *Physical Therapy*, 87(9): 1132–1143.

Baum, F. (2007) Cracking the nut of health equity: Top down and bottom up pressure for action on the social determinants of health. *IUHPE Promotion and Education*, 14(2): 90–95.

Baum, F. (2008) *The New Public Health*. 3rd edition. Oxford: Oxford Higher Education.

Bernier, N. (2007) Health promotion program resilience and policy trajectories: A comparison of three provinces. In M. O'Neill et al. (eds) *Health Promotion in Canada: Critical Perspectives*. Toronto: Canadian Scholars' Press Inc, 1–11.

Berridge, V. (2007) Public health activism. *British Medical Journal*, 335: 1310–1312.

Bhattacharya, K., Winch, P., LeBan, K. and Tien, M. (2001) Community Health Workers. Incentives and disincentives: How they affect motivation, retention and sustainability. The Basic Support for Institutionalizing Child Survival Project (BASICS II). United States Agency for International Development (USAID), Arlington, Virginia.

Bjaras, G., Haglund, B. J. A. and Rifkin, S. (1991) A new approach to community participation evaluation. *Health Promotion International* 6(3): 1999–2006.

Boveldt, N., Vernooij-Dassen, M., Leppink, I., Samwel, H., Vissers, K. and Engels, Y. (2014) Patient empowerment in cancer pain management: An integrative literature review. *Journal of the Psychological, Social and Behavioral Dimensions of Cancer*, 23(11): 1203–1211.

Britten, N. (1995) Qualitative interviews in medical research. *British Medical Journal*, 311: 251–253.

Brown, P. and Zavestoski, S. (2004) Social movements in health: An introduction. *Sociology of Health & Illness*, 26(6): 679–694.

Brown, P., Zavestoski, S., McCormick, S., Mayer, B., Morello-Frosch, R. and Gasior, R. (2004) Embodied health movements: Uncharted territory in social movement research. *Sociology of Health & Illness*, 26(1): 50–80.

Burgess, R. G. (1982) *Field Research: A Source Book and Field Manual*. London: Allen & Unwin.

Cass, A., Lowell, A., Christie, M., Snelling, P. L., Flack, M., Marrnganyin, B. and Brown, I. (2002) Sharing the true stories: Improving communication between Aboriginal patients and health care workers. *The Medical Journal of Australia*, 176(10): 466–470.

Centre for Disease Control and Prevention (2006) Recommendations for future efforts in community health promotion. Regional expert panel on community health promotion, CDC, Atlanta, USA.

Cherkezova, S. and Tomova, I. (2013) An option of last resort? Migration of Roma and non-Roma from CEE countries. Roma inclusion working papers. UNDP Europe. Bratislava Regional Office.

Chewning, B., Bylund, C., Shah, B., Arora, N. K., Gueguen, J. A. and Makoul, G. (2012) Patient preferences for shared decisions: A systematic review. *Patient Education and Counseling*, 86(1): 9–18.

Chow, J., Murry, S. and Angeli, C. (1996) International and multicultural teaming: A kaleidoscope of kolors. Annual conference of the American Evaluation Association, Atlanta, Indiana University.

Christakis, N. A. and Fowler, J. H. (2007) The spread of obesity in a large social network over 32 years. *New England Journal of Medicine*, 357(4): 370–379.

Coleman, P. T. (2000) Power and conflict. In Deutsch, M. and Coleman, P. T. (eds) *The Handbook of Conflict Resolution. Theory and Practice*. San Francisco, CA: Jossey-Bass Publishers.

Commonwealth of Australia (2000) *Promoting Practical Sustainability*. Canberra: AusAID.

Confederation of British Industry (2006) Transforming Local Services. Confederation of British Industry Brief, London, July 2006.

CORE Group (2005) 'Scale' and 'Scaling-Up': A CORE Group Background Paper on 'Scaling-Up' Maternal, Newborn and Child Health Services. Washington, DC: The World Bank, July 2005.

Crondahl, K. and Karlsson, L. (2015) Roma empowerment and social inclusion through work-integrated learning. SAGE Open, January–March 2015, 1–10.

Crondahl, K., Karlsson, L. and Eklund-Karlsson, L. (2015) Work-integrated learning and health literacy – catalysts for Roma empowerment and social inclusion? PhD thesis. Section 4. Unit for Health Promotion Research. University of Southern Denmark, Submitted 2014.

D'Agostino, S. (2014) The missing piece: Empowerment of grassroots Roma organisations in EU Roma integration policies. Policy brief. 2014/10. Institute for European Studies, Brussels.

Dryden, W. and Feltham, C. (1993) *Brief Counselling: A Practical Guide for Beginning Practitioners*. Milton Keynes: Open University Press.

Earle, L., Fozilhujaev, B., Tashbaeva, C. and Djamankulova, K. (2004) Community development in Kazakhstan, Kyrgyzstan and Uzbekistan. Occasional Paper Number 40. Oxford: INTRAC.

Eklund-Karlsson, L., Crondahl, K., Sunnemark, F. and Andersson, Å. (2013) The meaning of health, well-being, and quality of life perceived by Roma people in West Sweden. *Societies*, 3(2): 243–260.

Equality (2015) Roma and empowerment. http://www.equality.uk.com accessed 22 May 2015.

Ewles, L. and Simnett, I. (2003) *Promoting Health. A Practical Guide*. 5th edition. London: Bailliere Tindall.

Eyerman, R. and Jamison, A. (1991) *Social Movements. A Cognitive Approach*. Cambridge: Polity Press.

Faulkner, M. (2001) Empowerment and disempowerment: Models of staff/patient interaction. *Nursing Times Research*, 6(6): 936–948.

Fitzpatrick, S., Schumann, K. and Hill-Briggs, F. (2013) Problem solving interventions for diabetes self-management and control: A systematic review of the literature. Diabetes *Research and Clinical Practice*, 100(2): 145–161.

Foucault, M. (1979) *Discipline and Punishment: The Birth of the Prison*. Middlesex: Peregrine Books.

Freire, P. (2005) *Education for Critical Consciousness*. New York: Continuum Press.

Gallarotti, G. (2011) Soft power: what is it, why is it important and the conditions for its effective use. *Journal of Political Power*, 4(1): 25–47.

Gangolli, L. V., Duggal, R. and Shukla, A. (eds) (2005) *Review of Health Care in India*. Mumbai: CEHAT.

Gibbon, M., Labonté, R. and Laverack, G. (2002) Evaluating community capacity. *Health and Social Care in the Community*, 10(6): 485–491.

Gilmore, G. (2011) *Needs and Capacity Assessment for Health Education and Health Promotion*. 4th edition. Boston, MA: Jones and Bartlett Learning.

Ginsberg, P. E. (1988) Evaluation in cross-cultural perspective. *Evaluation and Program Planning*, 11: 189–195.

Giuntoli, G., Kinsella, K. and South, J. (2012) *Evaluation of the 'Altogether Better' Asset Mapping in Sharrow and Firth Park, Sheffield*. Leeds, UK: Leeds Metropolitan University, Institute for Health and Wellbeing.

Glesne, C. and Peshkin, A. (1992) *Becoming Qualitative Researchers*. New York: Longman Publishing Group.

Goodman, R. M., Speers, M. A., McLeroy, K., Fawcett, S., Kegler, M., Parker, E., Rathgeb Smith, S., Sterling, T. D. and Wallerstein, N. (1998) Identifying and defining the dimensions of community capacity to provide a basis for measurement. *Health Education & Behavior*, 25(3): 258–278.

Haynes, A. W. and Singh, R. N. (1993) Helping families in developing countries: A model based on family empowerment and social justice. *Social Development Issues*, 15(1): 27–37.

Hayward, B. (2006) Public participation. In Miller, R. (ed.) *New Zealand Government and Politics*. Auckland, New Zealand: Oxford University Press, 514–524.

Health Promotion Agency New Zealand (2015) Active Healthy Strong Community Partnerships. www.hpa.org.nz accessed 3 February 2015.

Hunt, K. and Emslie, C. (2001) Commentary: The prevention paradox in lay epidemiology – Rose revisited. *International Journal of Epidemiology*, 30(3): 442–446.

Improvement Network (2011) Patient involvement. www.tin.nhs.uk/patient-involvement accessed 10 April 2015.

Israel, B. A., Checkoway, B., Schultz, A. and Zimmerman, M. (1994) Health education and community empowerment: Conceptualizing and measuring perceptions of individual, organisational and community control. *Health Education Quarterly*, 21(2): 149–170.

Jackson, T., Mitchell, S. and Wright, M. (1989) The community development continuum. *Community Health Studies*, 8(1): 66–73.

Jadad, A. and O'Grady, L. (2008) How should health be defined? *British Medical Journal, Editorial*, 337: a2900.

Jirojwong, S. and Liamputtong, P. (eds) (2009) *Population Health, Communities and Health Promotion*. London: Oxford University Press.

Johansen, E., Diop, N., Laverack, G. and Leye, E. (2013) What works and what does not: A discussion of popular approaches for the abandonment of female genital mutilation. *Obstetrics and Gynaecology International*, Advance access ID 348248: 1–10.

Jones, L. and Sidell, M. (eds) (1997) *The Challenge of Promoting Health. Exploration and Action*. London: Macmillan.

Kant, I., Gregor, M. and Reath, A. (1997) *Kant: Critique of Practical Reason*. Cambridge: Cambridge University Press.

Kendall, S. (1998) (ed.) *Health and Empowerment: Research and Practice*. London: Arnold.

Kettunen, T., Poskiparta, M. and Liimatainen, L. (2001) Empowering counselling – A case study: Nurse patient encounter in a hospital. *Health Education Research*, 16(2): 227–238.

Kieffer, C. H. (1984) Citizen empowerment: A development perspective. *Prevention in Human Services*, 3: 9–36.

Kitzinger, J. (1995) Introducing focus groups. *British Medical Journal*, 311: 299–302.

Klawiter, M. (2004) Breast cancer in two regimes: The impact of social movements on illness experience. *Sociology of Health & Illness*, 26(6): 845–874.

Kósa, K. and Adany, R. (2007) Studying vulnerable populations: Lessons from the Roma minority. *Epidemiology*, 18: 290–299.

Labonté, R. (1994) Health promotion and empowerment: Reflections on professional practice. *Health Education Quarterly*, 21(2): 253–268.

Labonté, R. (1998) A Community Development Approach to Health Promotion: A Background Paper on Practice Tensions, Strategic Models and Accountability Requirements for Health Authority Work on the Broad Determinants of Health. Edinburgh: Health Education Board for Scotland.

Labonté, R. and Laverack, G. (2008) *Health Promotion in Action: From Local to Global Empowerment*. London: Palgrave Macmillan.

The Lancet (2012) Patient empowerment – Who empowers whom? *The Lancet*, 379(9827): 1677.

Laverack, G. (1998) The concept of empowerment in a traditional Fijian context. *Journal of Community Health and Clinical Medicine for the Pacific*, 5(1): 26–29.

Laverack, G. (1999) Addressing the contradiction between discourse and practice in health promotion, unpublished PhD thesis. Melbourne: Deakin University.

Laverack, G. and Labonté, R. (2000) A planning framework for the accommodation of community empowerment goals within health promotion programming. *Health Policy and Planning*, 15(3): 255–262.

Laverack, G. (2001) An identification and interpretation of the organizational aspects of community empowerment. *Community Development Journal*, 36(2): 40–52.

Laverack, G. and Brown, K. M. (2003) Qualitative research in a cross-cultural context: Fijian experiences. *Qualitative Health Research*, 13(3): 1–10.

Laverack, G. (2004) *Health Promotion Practice: Power and Empowerment*. London: Sage Publications.

Laverack, G. (2007) *Health Promotion Practice: Building Empowered Communities*. London: Open University Press.

Laverack, G., 'Ofanoa, M., Nosa, V., Fa'alili, J. and Taufa, S. (2007) *Social and cultural perceptions of community empowerment in four Pacific Peoples in Auckland, New Zealand*. The University of Auckland, New Zealand.

Laverack, G. (2009) *Public Health: Power, Empowerment & Professional Practice*. 2nd edition. London: Palgrave Macmillan.

Laverack, G., Hill, K., Akenson, L. and Corrie, R. (2009) Building capacity towards health leadership in remote indigenous communities in Cape York. *Australian Indigenous Health Bulletin*, 9(1): 1–11.

Laverack, G. (2013) *Health Activism: Foundations and Strategies*. London: Sage Publications.

Laverack, G. (2014) *A to Z of Health Promotion*. Basingstoke: Palgrave Macmillan.

Laverack, G. (2015) *A to Z of Public Health*. London: Palgrave.

Lerner, M. (1986) *Surplus Powerlessness*. Oakland, CA: The Institute for Labour and Mental Health

Lindstrom, B. and Eriksson, M. (2005) Salutogenesis. *Journal of Epidemiology and Community Health*, 59(6): 440–442.

Lloyd, M. and Bor, R. (2004) *Communication Skills for Medicine*. 2nd edition. London: Churchill Livingstone.

Loss, J. and Wise, M. (2007) Concepts, benefits and limits of empowerment and participation in community based health promotion practice – Results of a qualitative study. Unpublished.

Lupton, D. (1995) *The Imperative of Health: Public Health and the Regulated Body*. London: Sage Publications.

MacPherson, D. W. and Gushulak, B. D. (2004) Global Migration Perspectives. Global Commission on International Migration. Geneva. Report Number 7. October 2004.

McAllister, M., Dunn, G., Payne, K., Davies, L. and Todd, C. (2012) Patient empowerment: The need to consider it as a measurable patient-reported outcome for chronic conditions. *BMC Health Services Research*, 12: 157.

Mackie, G. (1996) Ending footbinding and infibulation: A convention account. *American Sociological Review*, 61(6): 999–1017.

McLeod, J. and Mcleod, J. (2011) *A Practical Guide for Counsellors and Helping Professionals*. London: Open University Press.

Manandhar, D. S., Osrin, D., Prasad Shrestha, B., Mesko, N., Morrison, J., Tumbahanghe, K. M., Tamang, S., Thapa, S., Shrestha, D., Thapa, B., Shrestha, J. R., Wade, A., Standing, H., Manandhar, M., Costello, A. M. and members of the MIRA Makwanpur trial team. (2004) Effect of a participatory intervention with women's groups on birth outcomes in Nepal: Cluster-randomised controlled trial. *The Lancet*, 364: 970–979.

Marlatt, G. A. and Witkiewitz, K. (2010) Update on harm-reduction policy and intervention research. *Annual Review of Clinical Psychology*, 6: 591–606.

Marshall, G. (1998) *A Dictionary of Sociology*. London: Oxford University Press.

Martin, B. (2007) Activism, social and political. In Andersen, G. L. and Herr, K. G. (eds) *Encyclopedia of Activism and Social Justice*. London: Sage Publications.

Mason, M. (2010) Sample size and saturation in PhD studies using qualitative interviews [63 paragraphs]. *Forum Qualitative Sozialforschung/Forum: Qualitative Social Research*, 11(3): 1–8.

Minichiello, V., Aroni, R., Timewell, E. and Alexander, L. (1990) *Indepth Interviewing. Researching People*. Melbourne, Australia: Longman Cheshire.

Ministry of Health (2003) Project to Counter Stigma and Discrimination Associated with Mental Illness. National Plan 2003–2005. Wellington, New Zealand: Ministry of Health.

Ministry of Health and Ministry of Pacific Island Affairs (2004) *Tupu Ola Moui: Pacific Health Chart Book*. Wellington, New Zealand: Ministry of Health.

Mitchell, C. and Banks, M. (1998) *Handbook of Conflict Resolution. The Analytical Problem-Solving Approach*. London: Pinter.

Monti, P. M., Colby, S. M., Barnett, N. P., Spirito, A., Rohsenow, D. J., Myers, M., Woolard, R. and Lewander, W. (1999) Brief intervention for harm reduction and alcohol practices in older adolescents in a hospital emergency department. *Journal of Counselling and Clinical Psychology*, 76(6): 989–994.

Naidoo, J. and Wills, J. (2009) *Foundations of Health Promotion*. 3rd edition. London: Bailliere and Tindall.

National Health Service (2015) NHS values summit. www.england.nhs.uk accessed 18 April 2015.

NHS North West (2011) *Development of a Method for Asset Based Working*. Manchester: NHS North West and Department of Health.

Nutbeam, D. (2000) Health literacy as a public health goal: A challenge for contemporary health education and communication strategies into the 21st century. *Health Promotion International*, 15(3): 259–267.

O'Connor, M. and Parker, E. (1995) *Health Promotion: Principles and Practice in the Australian Context*. St Leonards, NSW: Allen & Unwin Pty Ltd.

Open Society Foundations (2012) Empowerment through Employment: Capitalizing on the Economic Opportunities of Roma Inclusion. Open Society Roma Initiatives policy brief. September 2012.

Pakulski, J. (1991) *Social Movements. The Politics of Moral Protest*. Sydney: Longman Cheshire.

Papa, M. J., Singhal, A. and Papa, W. H. (2006) *Organizing for Social Change: A Dialectic Journey of Theory and Praxis*. London: Sage Publications.

Patient Concern (2012) http://www.patientconcern.org.uk/ accessed 15 January 2012.

Patient UK (2012) www.patient.co.uk accessed 21 May 2012.

Patients Association (2015) http://www.patients-association.org.uk accessed 15 April 2015.

Perry, P. and Webster, A. (1999) *New Zealand Politics at the Turn of the Millennium*. Auckland, New Zealand: Alpha Publications.

Pescosolido, B. A. (1991) Illness Careers and Network Ties: A Conceptual Model of Utilization and Compliance. In Albrecht, G. and Levy, J. (eds) *Advances in Medical Sociology*. Greenwich, CT: JAI Press, 161–184.

PhotoVoice (2015) Social change through photography. www.photovoice.org accessed 31 March 2015.

Plows, A. (2007) Strategies and tactics in social movements. In Andersen, G. L. and Herr, K. G. (eds) *Encyclopedia of Activism and Social Justice*. London: Sage Publications.

Rappaport, J. (1985) The power of empowerment language. *Social Policy*, Fall: 15–21.

Raven, B. H. and Litman-Adizes, T. (1986) Interpersonal influence and social power in health promotion. In Ward, W. B. (ed.) *Advances in Health Education and Promotion*. London: Elsevier Science Ltd., 181–209.

Renkert, S. and Nutbeam, D. (2001) Opportunities to improve maternal health literacy through antenatal education: An explanatory study. *Health Promotion International*, 16(4): 381–388.

Rifkin, S. B., Muller, F. and Bichmann, W. (1988) Primary health care: On measuring participation. *Social Science Medicine*, 9: 931–940.

Rifkin, S. B. and Pridmore, P. (2001) *Partners in Planning: Information, Participation and Empowerment*. London: Macmillan Education.

Rifkin, S. (2006) Patient empowerment: Increased compliance or total transformation? 'Patient Empowerment'. In Porzolt, F. and Kaplan, R. (eds) *Optimizing Health: Improving the Value of Health Care Delivery*. Frankfurt: Springer, Chapter 9, 66–73.

Rissel, C. (1994) Empowerment: The holy grail of health promotion? *Health Promotion International*, 9(1): 39–47.

Ritter, A. and Cameron, J. (2006) A review of the efficacy and effectiveness of harm reduction strategies for alcohol, tobacco and illicit drugs. *Drug and Alcohol Review*, 25(6): 611–624.

Roberts, H. (1998) Empowering communities: The case of childhood accidents. In Kendall, S. (ed.) *Health and Empowerment: Research and Practice*. London: Arnold, Chapter 6.

Rosato, M., Laverack, G., Grabman, L. H., Tripathy, P., Nair, N., Mwansambo, C., Azad, K., Morrison, J., Bhutta, Z., Perry, H., Rifkin, S. and Costello, A. (2008) Alma Ata: Rebirth and revision 5: Community participation: Lessons for maternal, newborn and child health. *The Lancet*, 372(9642): 962–972.

Roughan, J. J. (1986) Village organization for development, PhD thesis. Honolulu, HI: Department of Political Science, University of Hawaii.

Russon, C. (1995) The influence of culture on evaluation. *Evaluation Journal of Australasia*, 7(1): 44–49.

Salmon, P. and Hall, G. M. (2004) Patient empowerment or the emperor's new clothes. *Journal of the Royal Society of Medicine*, 97(2): 53–56.

Saskatoon Regional Health Authority (SRHA) (2005) *Saskatoon 'In Motion': Five Years in the Making*. Saskatchewan: Saskatoon Regional Health Authority.

Scrambler, G. (1987) Habermas and the power of medical expertise. In Scrambler, G. (ed.) *Sociological Theory and Medical Sociology*. New York: Methuen Press, 50–55.

Seefeldt, F. M. (1985) Cultural considerations for evaluation consulting in the Egyptian context. In Patton, M. Q. (ed.) *Culture and Evaluation*. San Francisco, CA: Jossey-Bass, 69–78.

Seidman, S. and Wagner, D. G. (eds) (1992) *Postmodernism and Social Theory. The Debate Over General Theory*. Oxford: Blackwell.

Seiter, R. H. and Gass, J. S. (2010) Persuasion, *Social Influence, and Compliance Gaining*. 4th edition. Boston, MA: Allyn & Bacon.

Seligman, M. (1975) *Helplessness: On Depression, Development and Death*. San Francisco, CA: W. H. Freeman.

Simpson, G. E. and Yinger, J. M. (1965) *Racial and Cultural Minorities*. New York: Harper and Row.

Smith, R. (2002) The discomfort of patient power. *British Medical Journal*, 324: 497–498.

Smithies, J. and Webster, G. (1998) *Community Involvement in Health*. Aldershot, England: Ashgate Publishing Ltd.

South, J., White, J. and Gamsu, M. (2013) *People-Centred Public Health*. University of Bristol: Policy Press.

Srinivasan, L. (1993) *Tools for Community Participation. A Manual for Training Trainers in Participatory Techniques*. New York: PROWWESS/UNDP.

Starhawk, M. S. (1990) *Truth or Dare. Encounters with Power, Authority and Mystery*. New York: HarperCollins.

Stewart, M. A., Brown, J. B., Weston, W. W., et al. (2003) *Patient Centred Medicine: Transforming the Clinical Method*. 2nd edition. Oxford: Radcliffe Medical Publications.

Tengland, P. (2007) Empowerment: A goal or a means for health promotion? *Medicine, Health Care and Philosophy*, 10: 197–207.

Tidy, C. (2015) Patient groups. patient.co.uk accessed 1 February 2015.

Tomova, I. (2013) Good practices of Roma inclusion: Case studies in Bulgaria, Czech Republic and Belgium. In Cherkezova, S. and Tomova, I. (eds) *An Option of Last Resort? Migration of Roma and non-Roma from CEE Countries*. Roma inclusion working papers. UNDP Europe. Bratislava Regional Office.

Tse, S., Laverack, G., Nayar, S. and Foroughian, S. (2011) Community engagement for health promotion: Reducing injuries among Chinese people in New Zealand. *Health Education Journal*, 70(1): 76–83.

Turner, B. S. and Samson, C. (1995) *Medical Power and Social Knowledge*. London: Sage Publications.

UNAIDS (1999) *Peer education HIV/AIDS. Concepts, uses and challenges*. Geneva: UNAIDS.

UNICEF (2001) *Beyond Child Labour: Affirming Rights*. New York: UNICEF.

Uphoff, N. (1991) A field methodology for participatory self-education. *Community Development Journal*, 26(4): 271–285.

van Baar, H. (2011) Europe's Romaphobia: Problematization, securitization, nomadization. *Environment and Planning D: Society and Space*, 29: 203–212.

van Til, J. A., Drossaert, C. C., Renzenbrink, G. J., Snoek, G. J., Dijkstra, E., Stiggelbout, A. M. and IJzerman, M. J. (2010) Feasibility of web-based decision aids in neurological patients. *Journal of Telemedicine and Telecare*, 16(1): 48–52.

Volunteering England (2012) What is volunteering? www.volunteering.org.uk accessed 5 January 2015.

Walley, J., Wright, J. and Hubley, J. (2001) *Public Health: An Action Guide to Improving Health in Developing Countries*. Oxford: Oxford University Press.

Wang, C. C. and Pies, C. A. (2004) Family, maternal and child health through photovoice. *Maternal and Child Health Journal*, 8(2): 95–102.

Wanless, D. (2003) *Securing Good Health for the Whole Population: Population Health Trends*. London: HMSO.

Wartenberg, T. E. (1990) *The Forms of Power. From Domination to Transformation*. Philadelphia, PA: Temple University Press.

Weatherburn, D. (2009) Dilemmas in harm minimization. *Addiction*, 104(3): 335–339.

Werner, D. (1988) Empowerment and health: Contact. *Christian Medical Commission*, 102: 1–9.

Wharf-Higgins, J., Naylor, P. and Day, M. (2007) Seed funding for health promotion: Sowing sustainability or scepticism? *Community Development Journal*, 1–12. Advance access 31 January 2007.

White, H. C. (1992) *Identity and Control: A Structured Theory of Social Action*. Princeton, NJ: Princeton University Press.

Winfield, M. (2013) *The Essential Volunteer Handbook*. Victoria, BC: Friesen Press.

World Health Organization (1978) *Declaration of Alma Ata*. Geneva: World Health Organization.

World Health Organization (1986) *Ottawa Charter for Health Promotion*. Geneva: World Health Organization.

World Health Organization (1998) *Health Promotion Glossary*. Geneva: World Health Organization.

World Health Organization (2007a) *Operationalising Empowerment to Improve Maternal and Newborn Health: A Guide to the Workshop for Maternal and Newborn Health Programme Managers and Providers*. Geneva: World Health Organization (unpublished report).

World Health Organization (2007b) *Health of Indigenous Peoples*. Fact sheet number 326. Geneva: World Health Organization.

Wright, E. R. (1997) The impact of organizational factors on mental health professionals' involvement with families. *Psychiatric Services*, 48: 921–927.

Wrong, D. H. (1988) *Power. Its Forms, Bases and Uses*. Chicago, IL: The University of Chicago Press.

Zakus, J. D. L. and Lysack, C. L. (1998) Revisiting community participation. *Health Policy and Planning*, 13(1): 1–12.

# INDEX